CHRONIC ILLNESS
AND
UNCERTAINTY

CHRONIC ILLNESS AND UNCERTAINTY

A PERSONAL AND PROFESSIONAL GUIDE TO POORLY UNDERSTOOD SYNDROMES

What We Know And Do Not Know About Fibromyalgia, Chronic Fatigue, Migraine, Depression and Related Illnesses

Don L. Goldenberg M.D.
Dorset Press
PO Box 620026
Newton Lower Falls, MA 02162

Library of Congress Cataloging-in-Publication Data
Goldenberg, Don
  Chronic Illness and Uncertainty, 1996
  Number: 96-92858

ISBN: 0-9656102-0-9

Published by Dorset Press
PO Box 620026
Newton Lower Falls, MA 02162

For Patty,
my inspiration and my love

CONTENTS

ACKNOWLEDGMENTS

First, I would like to thank the thousands of patients who have helped me learn about chronic illness. Many have been truly heroic.

Next, I want to thank my professional colleagues, especially those who have shared my interest in fibromyalgia, chronic fatigue and related disorders. Many from around the world are mentioned in the book or in the references and notes section. Some, like Dr Joanne Borg-Stein, Dr Ken Kaplan and Maureen Nadeau, have worked closely with me during the past decade.

A special thanks to my editor, Lucy D. Phillips. Her insight and style sharpened the focus of what I wanted to convey. My good friend, Ken Dreyer, was my "sounding-board" and my most helpful critic. My office staff, including Chris Mossey and Janine Beauchemin, spent hours helping with the book preparation and organizing my activities so that I could find time for this project.

During my own recent illnesses, Dr Mike Levin, my primary care physician, and the medical and nursing staff at Newton-Wellesley Hospital gave me great medical care. Dr Nick Browning has been an immeasurable source of comfort, education and encouragement.

Finally, I most want to thank my wife and wonderful family for their love and support during the good times and the bad.

INTRODUCTION

We have all felt pain and stiffness in our muscles, pain in our backs, headaches, abdominal pain, and bowel irregularity. Most of us have felt exhaustion, anxiety, or depression, often accompanied by sleep problems. Generally, these episodes are transient, or short-lived. They usually follow a precipitating factor, a recognizable cause such as physical injury, infection, or emotional upheaval.

However, 10-20 percent of the population suffers from one or more of these symptoms for months or even years at a time. Often a precipitating factor is lacking or long forgotten in the past. Since we have a population of 250 million, that means 25 to 50 million Americans are living with chronic muscle and back pain, chronic fatigue, headaches, insomnia, bowel irritability, depression and other mood disturbances.

These chronic problems often occur simultaneously. Why they become chronic and why they occur together in so many of us is a mystery to me and my medical colleagues. In medical jargon, they are "poorly understood," yet we affix diagnostic labels: fibromyalgia, chronic fatigue syndrome, irritable bowel syndrome, migraine, insomnia and depression.

This book discusses all of these conditions because both doctors and patients need to understand them better.

It concentrates on fibromyalgia and chronic fatigue because they have been the focus of my own practice and research.

My reasons for writing the book are both professional and personal. Professionally, I am concerned by the opposing and often hostile views voiced by physicians and the public about these disorders. The medical profession often discards them as fads or signs of psychological distress. Others consider that chronic pain and fatigue are simply a part of normal life. They declare that pasting a diagnostic label on symptoms we all have, at one time or another, promotes a "sick role." Even physicians who sympathetically treat patients with these illnesses do not know whether the mind or the body is primarily at fault. In short, confusion and uncertainty abound in the diagnosis and management of these disorders.

In direct contrast to skeptical and puzzled physicians, some groups of health care professionals or patients claim to know the causes and treatment of chronic pain, fatigue or headaches. They are convinced that such disorders result from infections, immune abnormalities, foods or environmental toxins. Unfounded reports of remedies and cures pop up in self-help books. Their mostly well-meaning authors have carved out their own turf and cling to their beliefs. They are often mistrustful of traditional medicine, just as traditional physicians tend to mistrust "alternative medicine."

Since the medical profession lacks clear understanding and direction with regard to these problems, patients not surprisingly turn to alternative sources for information and treatment, especially when these sources claim to have the answers.

My hope in writing this book is to provide a bridge and balance between the professional and public views of these disorders. I cannot reveal their exact cause or offer a magic cure. But I can help the reader to understand how they interrelate, share symptoms, and—perhaps most important—how their very uncertainties increase their negative impact. Whether defined as a disease or a syndrome, they cause illness. Illness is made worse by uncertainty, so understanding will help.

Books have already been written on each of these disorders: fibromyalgia, chronic back pain, chronic fatigue syndrome, insomnia, migraine, irritable bowel syndrome and depression. But while they seek to set each disorder apart, this book will highlight their many similarities. I believe that understanding the common nature of these syndromes is much more important than describing their uniqueness. They are linked to one another, and people who suffer from any one of them will very likely turn up with another as well. These syndromes share a basic pathology that involves both our minds and our bodies. Each is plagued by diagnostic and therapeutic uncertainty.

My personal reasons for writing this book include my wife's long battle with fibromyalgia. As a rheumatologist, my patients almost always have a chronic and painful problem. Many are poorly understood, like rheumatoid arthritis or systemic lupus erythematosus, and can only be managed, not cured. These patients and their problems are important and compelling, but I have also focused much of my time and effort on fibromyalgia since I discovered it to be the root of my own wife's struggle. She is now living well with her symptoms, and I have become one of the country's leading experts on fibromyalgia. For the past 20 years I have listened to and worked with thousands of patients with fibromyalgia, as well as chronic pain, fatigue and depression. I have directed a number of related research studies.

An even more personal reason for the book is my own experience of chronic health problems. In my adult life I've had, like many people, a number of serious medical problems. They include poorly understood chronic pain, debilitating headaches, profound exhaustion, terrible insomnia, anxiety and depression. Looking back, I recognize a "domino effect," with one leading quite naturally to the next. But as each came along, I was a typical worried and frustrated patient, despite being a physician.

After all, physicians are humans who get sick like everyone else. In fact, while medical training has advantages in coping with ones own illness, it also has disadvantages. As I suffered my series of problems, I kept thinking, "I can deal with this. I can handle stress, pain, and uncertainty. After all, this is what I do for a living! This is what I was trained to do." So I felt excessive frustration when I lost control over the very symptoms that I had been researching and treating in others. My professional experience and knowledge did not help me to cope with uncertain diagnosis and treatment.

In short, chronic illness and its uncertainty have been persistent themes in my life and in my career. To this book I bring the insight of an insider (the patient) and an outsider (the physician). I've tried to write a "physician's guide" to coping with these illnesses that offers a "patient's view" of their uncertainty and frustration. I share experiences from my medical practice, my wife's battle with fibromyalgia, and the puzzles of my own health.

The book is divided into four sections. Section I is devoted to fibromyalgia and chronic fatigue. Section II discusses common illnesses that are often associated, including chronic back pain, insomnia, migraine and other headaches, irritable bowel, intellect and memory disturbances and depression. Section III explores the public (and patients') view of these illnesses and the often opposite view of the traditional medical profession. The conflicting perceptions of patients and their physicians must not be shrugged off or ridiculed. They need to be recognized and reconciled. Each side has contributions to make. Finally,

Section IV discusses ways to best manage these chronic illnesses, their uncertainty and their symptoms.

If you are interested in a succinct "how-to" approach, you may wish to focus on the last section. But I believe understanding is important, and understanding requires the in-depth discussion covered by Sections I through III. Whatever your focus, the book allows you to follow the narrative alone or to utilize, in addition, the extensive annotated bibliography and appendix with tables and figures. This material can provide a more detailed medical and scientific background for those who are interested.

When you finish this book, you will have a better broad picture of chronic illnesses and a better handle on living with each of them. You will also understand and accept better the uncertainty inherent in fibromyalgia, chronic fatigue and associated illnesses, as well as the uncertainty of our health in general.

SECTION I:
FIBROMYALGIA AND CHRONIC FATIGUE SYNDROME

Chapter 1:
Disease, illness, and syndromes

N othing causes us greater concern than our health and the health of those we love. The greater our uncertainty about a disease or illness, the greater our concern.

Disease and illness are not the same thing, though the words are often used interchangeably. A disease is a disorder of an organ, organ system, or body part. Illness is the interaction of our mind and body with our surroundings. It is defined in terms of how a particular disorder affects a particular individual. For example, a heart attack is seen most simply as something wrong with the heart—the acute sign of chronic heart disease. However, the associated illness is much more complicated. It results from the impact of disease on the individual, and this varies with many factors.

Health problems can be classified into three broad categories based on the level of uncertainty involved for both physician and patient (Table 1). In the first category are disorders with a clear cause and scientific basis. If you break a bone, the acute pain you feel is easy to understand. Treatment is straight-forward and recovery is usually gradual but complete. Similarly, infectious diseases like the common cold, pneumonia and tuberculosis are easy to understand. These diseases are generally diagnosed quickly and exactly. Treatment is often very specific, such as an antibiotic that can kill the microorganism causing the problem. However, even when we know the cause, we often do not know why a particular person gets a particular disease. The choice of therapy, individual disease course, or length of time to recovery are other questions. But uncertainty is relatively minimal in this first category.

In the second category are a large number of diseases for which the pathology and physiology are at least partly understood, but for which a single cause has not been identified. They are often chronic or recurrent diseases that are managed rather than completely cured. Good examples are heart disease, high blood pressure, chronic lung disease, cancer, stroke, and many of the immunologic disorders like rheumatoid arthritis, systemic lupus erythematosus (lupus), and multiple sclerosis. Their etiology—their cause and development—is widely accepted to involve interaction of the host (our genetic makeup) and the environment (what we eat, inhale, or what we are infected with). Many host and environmental factors influence the disease expression; course and treatment vary greatly. So this category of disease has significant elements of uncertainty and lack of understanding.

People can react very differently when struck by the same kind of disease calamity, as shown by the two cases that follow.

Alan and Steve: two heart attacks

Alan, a 55-year-old attorney, had a heart attack three years ago. He is a very successful lawyer who became a full partner in a large Boston firm at age 35. He had always worked a very demanding schedule, putting in an average of 60-70 hours weekly. He described himself as a type A personality. He had a family history of heart disease. His father had a heart attack at age 45. He also reported that he would hold everything inside, but then "blow up" and lose his temper at least once a month. He became more and more annoyed with inconveniences and "incompetence" and found himself frequently losing his temper when driving from the suburbs into Boston. Two months before his heart attack, he consulted with me because of persistent fatigue. His complete medical evaluation was unremarkable, but his cholesterol level was 350, more than twice the ideal value.

When I first saw him in the hospital 4 days after his heart attack, he was in good spirits. He told me that the heart attack was "a blessing in disguise" since it had given him the chance to reflect on his life and career. Having no financial worries, he planned on taking the next 3 months off, then resuming his work schedule at a much more leisurely pace. Indeed, he took off the following 2 months and also stopped smoking. He began to exercise regularly and felt much more relaxed. However, within 6 months he was back to his previous work schedule, not exercising and smoking again. When I talked to him about the dangers of his lifestyle, he projected a lot of denial. He once again was arguing with other drivers when coming and going from work. He became even more demanding of his employees and his family. He again began to have chest pain, but refused to acknowledge it to himself or his physicians. That is, until his second heart attack this past year. Currently, he is having difficulty coping with his heart disease and is unwilling to make major changes in his work and lifestyle.

Steve is a 59-year-old, 6-foot, 250-pound factory worker who had a number of severe sports and work injuries which resulted in arthritis of his right hip and left knee. He had consulted with me about his arthritis. Because of his arthritis, he had stopped jogging a few years ago. When he stopped exercising, he gained 40 pounds. He had a "mild heart attack" last year. When I visited with him shortly after the heart attack, he was very depressed and anxious. At first he was unable to open up to me about his concerns. However, after some probing, he told me that he felt a loss of his masculinity and was worried about his ability to support his family. At home he became immobilized with fear about resuming normal daily activities. He could not have normal sexual relations with his wife because of his fears of provoking another heart attack.

We enrolled him in a cardiovascular fitness training program. This included carefully structured stationary biking and water exercises. He gradually felt more confident as he became more active. His rehabilitation program also included counseling about how people respond to having a serious illness. This was very helpful to the patient and to his wife. He also gradually changed to a low-fat diet and cut down markedly on his beer intake. Currently, he is having no pain nor other medical problems. He recently told me that he feels alive again and he feels proud of the adjustments that he has made in his life.

Some risk factors for disease are beyond our control. Alan had a strong family history of heart disease and an elevated cholesterol count, both genetically predetermined. But Alan's response to his disease—or, more accurately, his *illness*—was very different than Steve's. How we react to a life-threatening event, like a heart attack, may have as much to do with the outcome as do our genetics or the severity of our disease.

Alan knew the importance of making life-style changes to help prevent future cardiac decompensation. He knew he was a type A personality. He was aware that research has documented that mental stress causes heart ischemia (lowered blood supply) and that this is associated with a greater risk of heart attacks (1). He knew that modification of the stress response has been shown to reduce the risk of future cardiac catastrophes (2). However, after a temporary effort, he could not change the patterns of his diet, exercise, and work habits. He was unable to relax and thus continued in his exaggerated stress reaction to the daily annoyances of life.

In contrast, Steve was at first less knowledgeable or motivated than Alan, but ultimately more able to change. Once past the fear of returning to normal activities, he gradually made major adjustments that involved regular exercise and a better diet. Initially he needed reassurance that he could resume sexual activities with his wife. We discussed research studies showing a one-in-a-million chance that sexual activity can trigger a heart attack (2). The switch from normal to sexual exertion is hardly more shocking to our system than our daily switch from sleeping to waking.

Individual reactions to illness are most important in the third category of medical problems. Often called syndromes (Table 1), these are health issues that cannot be neatly categorized as acute or chronic disease. They are medically defined as a group of signs and symptoms that adversely impact our health. To physicians, "signs" are the objective findings of careful examination whereas "symptoms" are reported by patients, and thus more subjective. Most syndromes are diagnosed by a patient's symptoms (Tables 2,3). Syndromes may cause chronic *illness* despite no clear *disease*. Their cause and pathology are not known. However, from one person to the next, their manifestations are reproducible. That is, their signs and symptoms occur repeatedly and consistently over time.

Syndromes—including fibromyalgia and chronic fatigue—are difficult to diagnose because there are no telltale physical or laboratory abnormalities (Table 3). Lacking objective evidence for "disease," their existence as specific entities is controversial. Such disorders are often termed "functional" because no structural or biochemical cause has been found. Many physicians are unfamiliar with their diagnostic criteria, so patients may go undiagnosed for years, whether they stay with one physician or desperately try many in succession. Even when syndromes are diagnosed and given sympathetic attention, there is no highly effective treatment.

Of the three categories of health problems, uncertainty is clearly the greatest with syndromes. In spite (or perhaps because) of this, the ten most common medical conditions are best classified as syndromes (Table 2). They include migraine and other chronic headaches, chronic low back pain, certain joint and muscle conditions like fibromyalgia, allergies, insomnia, high blood pressure, digestive problems (e.g., irritable bowel syndrome), anxiety, and clinical depression (3). Though not disease in the classic biomedical sense, all these conditions have clear symptoms. For example, those of clinical depression include one or more of the following: persistent despair, hopelessness, isolation, mental confusion or lack of concentration, and lack of pleasure in activities that previously were pleasurable (Table 4).

These poorly understood complaints—suffered by virtually all of us at one time or another—often coexist or develop "hand in hand" in a person. They have many more similarities than differences, though each has a distinctive cardinal symptom (Table 3). The defining symptom of fibromyalgia is chronic, generalized muscle pain. In chronic fatigue syndrome (CFS), it is debilitating fatigue. In irritable bowel syndrome, it is the abdominal pain and alternating constipation and diarrhea.

The similarities and overlap among these syndromes are very striking. People with any one of them commonly complain of fatigue, muscle and joint pain, headaches, sleep disturbances, difficulty concentrating, irritability, and depression. Though the syndromes are largely chronic and last months or years, the physical examination is frustratingly "normal." Laboratory tests and x-rays also give normal results, and are performed mainly to rule out other disorders.

These syndromes are quite common. They affect 5 to 20 percent of the population, a wide range that reflects their controversial diagnosis. For reasons as yet unclear, they are more common in women than in men.

Until recently, traditional medicine in the United States paid little attention to these disorders. Since they are not life-threatening, they are even described as "benign." The classic medical model of cause and effect (seen most obviously in infection) does not fit. Many physicians—and even patients who suffer with these syndromes—think of symptoms like headaches or anxiety as simply part of daily life, not "pathologic." Many patients even feel defensive or somehow to blame for their symptoms, which only magnifies their illness.

There has been a long debate in medicine as to whether these syndromes are primarily physical or psychological entities. In all of them, the mechanism of illness follows a similar pathway that involves a complicated *interaction* of mind and body (Figure 1). Such interaction is present, in varying degree, even in many diseases widely considered strictly physical, such as rheumatoid arthritis. And when the mind is a major factor, this does not automatically make a disease "all in the mind." It is no less legitimate or real.

Because of such complications, no single branch of medicine has taken the lead in understanding and treating many of these disorders. Good examples of such illnesses are fibromyalgia and CFS, which I have been studying for the past twenty years.

Chapter 2:
Fibromyalgia

My personal and professional interest in fibromyalgia began when my wife Patty became ill in the late 1970s. Patty is the most upbeat, outgoing person I know—the kind who makes others feel good about themselves. But suddenly, in 1977, her normal energy and enthusiasm began to ebb away. She complained of severe aches and pains throughout her body. Her sleep became erratic and she awoke feeling exhausted.

She still looked healthy and had no signs of serious illness. Her doctors found no "medical cause" for her symptoms. So, since our children were small and I probably wasn't helping enough at home, my first thought was that she had slipped into a short-term clinical depression. As explained in Chapter 9, clinical depression is not simply having a "bad day" or a low mood. It is an acute or chronic illness that can occur, suddenly or gradually, when a person is overwhelmed by one major crisis or burdened with too many.

Clinical depression is common but did not apply in Patty's case. Her pain became more generalized and severe, which is rare with depression. Her pain was "all over," but would vary in localization and intensity. Her neck, shoulders, and upper back were especially painful.

Always an active person, she was too sore and tired to exercise. She had extreme tenderness in her muscles; her skin became very sensitive, and rashes developed.

Despite feeling exhausted, Patty could not sleep well. Pain often awoke her or kept her "half-awake" all night. It became a major struggle to get going in the morning. At the same time, she began experiencing marked dryness in her eyes and mouth. Her fingers and toes began to suffer cold sensitivity (called Raynaud's syndrome or phenomenon). Thinking she might have an immunologic illness, such as systemic lupus erythematosus (lupus), I sent her to a rheumatologist colleague. He suspected a disease of the connective tissues, such as lupus or scleroderma, but multiple blood tests and X-rays did not support this conclusion. Patty went to numerous other specialists who suspected either inflammation or an overactive immune response. They prescribed numerous anti-inflammatory or immunosuppressive drugs, none of which did any good.

She saw a neurologist because her muscle pain was associated with a peculiar numbness and tingling discomfort, primarily of the arms and legs. This can signal nerve irritation or pressure, as seen in carpal tunnel syndrome or a herniated disc. So Patty had an electromyogram and nerve conduction study. This painful test involves placement of electrodes around the extremities, then application of small electrical stimuli to see if the nerve conduction is normal. Again, results were inconclusive. However, a neuropathy around the elbows was suspected, so corticosteroids were injected into the ulnar nerve area at the elbow. This caused Patty plenty of pain but no improvement in her symptoms.

About that time, I found a medical article that discussed the fibromyalgia syndrome (4). As I read the article and began to research this illness, everything I read sounded just like Patty. Its cardinal symptom is all-over muscle pain and stiffness, plus "tender points." These are points of excessive tenderness at specific sites in the muscles, tendons, and ligaments. Other symptoms are profound fatigue, sleep disturbances, headaches, and bowel problems. Patients complain they never feel refreshed when they awake after sleep. But most distressing are the muscle and joint pains, which do not improve much with standard arthritis medications.

Fibromyalgia may develop soon after a stressful event, such as an injury, emotional trauma, or a severe flu (5) (Figure 1). But it often develops very gradually without any known or noticed precipitating factor. Criteria to make a diagnosis of fibromyalgia have now been established (6). They include diffuse or generalized body pain for at least three months, involving the trunk, arms and legs, plus the presence of at least 11 of 18 tender points (Table 3). The tender points come in pairs. They are found in anatomically vulnerable locations, where people often suffer common muscle strains, tendinitis, or bursitis: for example, the "tennis elbow" site. They are also found over locations painful in trochanteric bursitis of the hip and bursitis of the knee. The 18 tender points (9 pairs) that confirm a diagnosis of fibromyalgia represent its most commonly painful sites, but various other muscles and tendons may also be sore (Figure 2). An experienced physician must examine these areas, as well as the characteristic tender points, when considering the diagnosis of fibromyalgia.

As explained in the prior chapter, fibromyalgia is a typical syndrome in having no definitive physical examination features, blood tests, or x-ray findings. Therefore, its diagnosis depends on observing a patient's symptoms over time while systematically ruling out other illnesses.

The physician considers and excludes other causes of generalized pain mainly by taking a careful history and performing a detailed physical examination (7). Sometimes laboratory or x-ray testing is also required.

When a patient has suffered pain and fatigue for only a few months, the physician may suspect a chronic infection like infectious mononucleosis ("mono") or a more serious disease like rheumatoid arthritis. Either could initially present with no symptoms other than fatigue and generalized pain, like fibromyalgia. But unlike fibromyalgia, rheumatoid arthritis rapidly causes structural damage that is readily detected during physical examination. Physical findings, as well as x-ray findings, also identify—and rule out—degenerative diseases of the nervous system, such as multiple sclerosis.

When pain and fatigue have been present for months or years—without causing any structural damage—a disease is not likely to be present. In other words, the longer someone has had the characteristic symptoms of generalized pain and fatigue *without receiving a disease diagnosis*, the more likely he or she is to have fibromyalgia and/or chronic fatigue syndromes.

Unfortunately, even when months or years have elapsed, physicians may miss the diagnosis because they are not trained to think about these syndromes. They do not know the diagnostic criteria. They are unaware of "tender points" or exactly how to find and touch them. Any place becomes a "tender point" if the physician presses soft tissues too hard!

Diagnostic confusion is especially common when fibromyalgia begins in a localized fashion. For example, pain on just one side of the head and neck, or in the lower back, may suggest an orthopedic or neurologic problem. Confusion also arises when pain is regional. Some physicians then diagnose myofascial pain syndrome, which they distinguish from fibromyalgia on the basis of "trigger points." Whereas tender points register pain only at the site of pressure, these points refer (or trigger) pain some distance down the limb. However, not all specialists distinguish fibromyalgia from myofascial pain, or tender points from trigger points.

Even when pain is generalized, fibromyalgia may be missed. It can be confused with infections, endocrine disorders, or immune disorders, and may even occur along with them. It is particularly likely to accompany lupus or rheumatic disorders like rheumatoid arthritis. However, patients with rheumatoid arthritis always show swelling and inflammation in their joints, which is not present in fibromyalgia. Patients with lupus usually have joint swelling as well as a characteristic rash. Both lupus and RA often cause inflammatory abnormalities in many organs, all revealed by various blood tests. (Speaking of tests, fibromyalgia can be accompanied by hypothyroidism, so thyroid function blood tests should always be performed.)

Patty had irritability of the bladder, dry eyes and mouth, and cold sensitivity. She also had paresthesias: numbness and tingling in her extremities. All of these symptoms hinder diagnosis of fibromyalgia since the first group can signal a systemic connective tissue disease, while paresthesias can signal a neurologic disorder.

Like Patty, fibromyalgia patients are often misdiagnosed as having a systemic rheumatic disease like lupus (8) or a neurologic disease like multiple sclerosis (9). Because so many conditions must be ruled out, even physicians experienced with fibromyalgia may need time to nail down the diagnosis. Patients improve their chances by selecting a physician who sees many patients with this illness. He or she is less likely to be fooled, having experienced all the diagnostic nuances and dilemmas of this elusive syndrome. Physicians lacking this experience can be like the fabled blind men describing their first elephant. One hugs a huge leg and says the animal must be like a tree. One grabs the tail and argues it must be like a rope, and so on. Generally, rheumatologists have the most experience with fibromyalgia, although it can also be diagnosed by primary care physicians, as well as physiatrists, neurologists, orthopedic surgeons, and other health care professionals.

Fibromyalgia syndrome, originally called fibrositis, was accurately described in the 1800s. However, the medical advances of the 20th century have brought limited progress. Since physical or laboratory examination show no major abnormalities, many doctors have considered it a wastebasket diagnosis or all in the head. Only in the last two decades has fibromyalgia begun to get respect among the medical profession.

I am proud to be one of the researchers who brought fibromyalgia into the medical mainstream. At the same time, I am humbled to admit that it took my own wife's illness to make me appreciate its seriousness. Seeing an illness up close, in someone you love and respect, changes your perspective. This woman with fibromyalgia was my wife. She wasn't crazy; she wasn't a hypochondriac. I had been taught that fibromyalgia, headaches, back pain, and chronic fatigue were non-specific symptoms, unworthy of scientific pursuit. They were certainly outside the realm of immunology and inflammatory arthritis, the backbone of my training and interests. But seeing them in Patty started me on a research mission. My practice began to include large numbers of patients with this and similar conditions.

My first step, in the early 1980s, was to discuss fibromyalgia with other interested physicians, and define its typical clinical manifestations. I was encouraged to find a number of highly respected clinicians who shared experiences with this perplexing illness: Rob Bennett, Fred Wolfe, Harvey Moldofsky, Hugh Smythe, Jon Russell, Muhammed Yunus, Sharon Clark, Carol Burckhardt,

Geoff Littlejohn, Karl Henriksson and many others throughout the world.

The most rewarding achievement of our collaboration has been the general recognition and acceptance by the medical profession of fibromyalgia as a discrete illness with its own set of symptoms and signs (6). In the early 1970s, when I did my training in rheumatology, fibromyalgia or fibrositis was simply ignored. My professors considered it to be a form of "psychogenic rheumatism." Now fibromyalgia is the second most frequent diagnosis that rheumatologists make in office practice (10). As clinical awareness has grown, medical school departments worldwide have joined the research pursuit to understand this illness.

In 1987, the prestigious and widely read *Journal of the American Medical Association* (JAMA) published my review of fibromyalgia (7). This helped to generate interest among physicians outside the specialty of rheumatology, including primary care physicians. Its title, "Fibromyalgia: An Emerging but Controversial Condition," turned out to be prophetic. The syndrome has indeed emerged as a well recognized and very common cause of chronic muscular pain and fatigue. The syndrome is generally accepted as the most common cause of chronic, diffuse pain in women between age 15 and 60. It is ten times more common in women than men, and usually begins between the ages of 20-50. However, it affects all age groups, including children and the elderly: an estimated 6-10 million people in the United States (7). Yet among physicians and scientists, the syndrome is still controversial, as are all those discussed in this book (11).

My own research studies have so far taken three directions. All reflect my fascination with the similarities between this syndrome, chronic fatigue syndrome, and the associated sleep and mood disturbances (Tables 3 and 4). We first investigated the view that fibromyalgia is a physical manifestation of depression. We found that most patients with fibromyalgia did not currently have major depression. However, we also found that these patients had more depression in their past, or in their family history, than did patients with other chronic rheumatic diseases, such as rheumatoid arthritis (Table 5) (12-15). This suggested a biologic link between fibromyalgia syndrome and mood disturbances. We therefore investigated the use of antidepressant medications to treat fibromyalgia, thinking that patients would benefit from their effect on serotonin and other neurotransmitters. Since our patients were seldom clinically depressed, we used very low doses of antidepressant medications—not high enough to treat depression. These low doses appeared to bring some improvement in pain, fatigue and sleep disturbances (16,17) (See Chapter 14: Medications).

Second, with scientists such as Tony Komaroff, Rob Simms, Dedra Buchwald and Jim Hudson, I have further explored the overlap of fibromyalgia with other chronic illnesses, especially chronic fatigue syndrome (CFS). We found that most CFS patients meet the criteria for the diagnosis of fibromyalgia (Table 6), (15,18,19). We also found that 50-70% of patients with fibromyalgia syndrome also suffered from migraine and irritable bowel syndrome (15,20). Our demonstration of these associations has helped bring together physicians who had focused on fibromyalgia or CFS, but not both. Each side has made contributions to the other, increasing progress for all.

Third and most recently, my research has turned to the brain and its neurotransmitters in relation to fibromyalgia and CFS. Investigators worldwide are exploring the role of the nervous system and the neurohormones that affect pain, sleep, mood and energy (21-23). In fibromyalgia, instead of looking for muscle abnormalities (24), we are looking for abnormalities in the central and peripheral nervous systems (21,22,25). Similar work is under way with regard to chronic fatigue, migraine, irritable bowel, and depression (5) (Figure 1).

Such research forms the basis of my approach to patients with fibromyalgia, but my wife's experience is also a major factor. I believe her illness has made me a better listener, a more empathetic physician who appreciates the "art" as well as the science of medicine. The art has to do with taking care of people, whether or not they can be cured. It has to do with helping them to understand and live with their illness. Patty's health problems and my own (mentioned in the next few chapters) have taught me to see the whole person when evaluating a patient.

My next challenge was to recognize that the most artful physician cannot offer all the training necessary to help patients with fibromyalgia. They need the care and expertise of an array of health professionals. They need a physician who is willing and able to coordinate a multidisciplinary treatment plan. We use many "physical" and "mental" health professionals and experts (Table 7). For example, for "hands on" physical treatment, I refer my fibromyalgia patients to a physiatrist. This physician—a specialist in physical medicine and rehabilitation—happens to offer special expertise in trigger point injections and acupuncture. Both are helpful in treating fibromyalgia, as detailed in Chapter 15. We also call on physical therapists, massage therapists, occupational therapists, podiatrists and other health care professionals, depending on individual patient needs.

Most of all, patients with fibromyalgia need information. Our first goal is to educate patients and their families to help them understand and cope with the illness. For each patient, the first office visit includes a 90-minute session to discuss what they are dealing with and what is likely to happen in the future. We talk about the intimate but mysterious relationship of the mind and body; the role of stress in pain, sleep, energy and adaptation to illness; the special difficulties that accompany an illness of uncertain diagnosis and therapy (for example the problems of dealing with skeptical relatives and physicians). Patients are encouraged to take an active role in their care, to be at the center of the treatment planning.

Our program includes medication, but we warn patients that medications will not always help. Often, a potentially helpful medication must be tailored to the individual. This can take time and patience. As with all aspects of treating fibromyalgia, trial and error is the *modus operandi*. Ideally, treatment should integrate medicinal (17,26) and non-medicinal therapies, as discussed in Section IV (27-29). The most helpful medications, so far, are those that interact with central nervous system chemicals such as serotonin and noradrenaline. For example, Patty has been taking very low bedtime doses of amitriptyline (Elavil) for much of the past 15 years. It helps to restore her deep sleep and relieve muscle pain and spasm.

Besides amitriptyline, patients with fibromyalgia have gained benefit from cyclobenzaprine and fluoxetine (Prozac) (17). They feel better with gradually increased exercise, which helps to build strength and energy. Ultimately, they can benefit from stretching and gentle types of cardiovascular exercise, such as walking or water exercises.

There is not yet a cure for fibromyalgia. Most studies that have tracked patients for years report that even when chronic pain and fatigue are managed and perhaps alleviated, they do not disappear. However, the big picture is more optimistic than suggested by research studies, which are conducted at tertiary care centers. These are metropolitan medical and research centers that tend to attract the sickest patients. Their symptoms have resisted treatment by their primary physician and community hospital. They have often seen several local physicians before coming to the tertiary center. Sometimes they have been mishandled by physicians, but often they simply have a tougher (more *resistant*) form of fibromyalgia. In contrast, "community patients" with perhaps milder forms of fibromyalgia can often benefit more from advice and medicines and often become symptom-free after a few months or years (30).

In my own practice, the vast majority of patients have improved. Most are working full-time, most do exercise, and most have adapted to their chronic illness with considerable equanimity. The typical patient with fibromyalgia can look forward to this kind of improvement. However, management of fibromyalgia is a "high maintenance" proposition! It demands a lot of work and patience from the physician, the patient, and patients' families. Everybody must be able to roll with the ups and downs of this chronic illness. Yet surely, as research unravels the mystery of fibromyalgia in the near future, we will have more effective weapons to fight this frustrating syndrome.

Chapter 3:
Chronic Fatigue Syndrome

About 6 months into my internship in a New York City hospital, I started to feel extremely tired. I attributed this to the rigors of training, but it evolved into a three-month bout of debilitating fatigue—the kind of exhaustion that makes it impossible to function normally. After the first month, I went to see one of the staff physicians. Blood tests found signs pointing to infectious mononucleosis. However, the tests for mono were not positive and my physician was puzzled.

This was my first encounter with a chronic and poorly understood illness. It was also my first experience with being *ill* but not being diagnosed with a *disease*.

People who work in medicine tend to fear developing one of the serious illnesses that they see around them every day. I wondered if I had lymphoma or leukemia. Fortunately, after some time off, I began to feel better and gradually returned to my old self. However, each year after that I would suffer a week or two of this profound fatigue. It would usually be diagnosed as the flu, but always seemed to last longer than flu lasts in most people.

These episodes made me appreciate the distress that profound and unexplained fatigue causes people. My experience would later pique my interest in better understanding chronic fatigue in my patients.

Fatigue is one of the most common complaints that brings people to a physician's office. Now and then, everyone has a day or two of fatigue, but 15-20 percent of the American population suffers chronic fatigue lasting for months at a time (31). It usually stems from a medical or psychiatric disease like depression, thyroid deficiency, anemia, arthritis, or immune disorders. But about 10 percent of these people have no apparent disease. Their ill-defined chronic fatigue has been given various names during the past century, most currently chronic fatigue syndrome (CFS).

What exactly is fatigue? In physiologic terms, it is defined as the failure to sustain an expected physical force (32). It can be objectively measured, as with a Cybex machine. However, when most of us complain of fatigue, we describe a more subjective feeling of tiredness or exhaustion. Until very recently, this pervasive sense of fatigue has not been measurable or well defined (32).

Yet inexplicable fatigue is not new to medicine. Old novels are full of mysteriously unwell female (and sometimes male) characters described as "neurasthenic." In the early 1900s, the physician George Beard coined the term *neurasthenia* to describe the "nervous exhaustion" reported by his patients with chronic fatigue (33). He popularized the notion that such fatigue was caused by a breakdown of the nervous system. Previously, neurasthenia or "the vapors" was often attributed to some kind of infection.

Over the next 50 years, cases of chronic, unexplained fatigue occurred in several epidemics (34-36). Large outbreaks were reported from Los Angeles, Iceland, South Africa, England, Australia, and other countries (37). The widespread nature of these cases suggested an infectious agent. The polio virus was then rampant, and many medical investigators suspected that an atypical form of polio was the culprit. However, no infection or fever could be found in the vast majority of the patients, and no patients died.

Many more women than men suffered this severe fatigue. In addition to exhaustion, patients generally had chronic muscle pain, or myalgias, and very tender muscles. The muscle pain was identical to that much later described in patients with fibromyalgia. Headaches, numbness and tingling of the limbs, memory and mood disturbances were common. In contrast to polio or most other infections that attack the nervous system, the illness never involved paralysis or muscle atrophy.

In the mid-20th century this illness was labeled *benign myalgic encephalomyelitis* (BME), *benign* meaning no deaths occurred, *myalgic* describing muscle pain, and *encephalomyelitis* suggesting a cause in the nervous system. The condition is still called BME in parts of the United Kingdom (38). Many patients experienced remissions and exacerbations of their symptoms for months or years. Flare-ups were often attributed to physical exertion, cold weather, or menstrual periods. Laboratory testing, x-rays, spinal taps, and muscle biopsies shed no light on the matter.

Since the medical profession could not prove that an infection or neurologic disease was present in BME or neurasthenia, some skeptics began to consider that this illness was psychosomatic. In its epidemic form, it was seen as a form of "mass hysteria," especially since mostly women were affected. (Interestingly, *hysteria* is a term rarely applied to men, perhaps because it comes from the Greek word for *uterus*.) Some epidemics, such as one reported from Los Angeles County Hospital, occurred almost exclusively in health care professionals. Cases were not uncommon in nurses taking care of patients with polio and other infectious diseases. Since there was no evidence for transmission of infection, it was postulated that their neurasthenia was caused by anxiety and fear of contagion (not to mention the grueling and demeaning conditions under which nurses then worked). Others held to the notion that these epidemics represented a new entity caused by an infection yet to be discovered (37).

In the early 1980s, a rash of cases was reported in which chronic fatigue seemed linked to the Epstein-Barr virus, agent of infectious mononucleosis (39). However, further research could not secure the link to the Epstein-Barr virus or any other single infection (40). Early hopes that a single cause for chronic fatigue would be found gradually faded in both patients and investigators, but particularly the latter. As mentioned later in this chapter, some patients came to feel betrayed by those researchers. Although a specific infection was not found, researchers slowly established the clinical features and diagnostic criteria for what we now call chronic fatigue syndrome (41,42). Its cardinal symptom is chronic, debilitating fatigue, but most patients also report muscle and joint pain, problems with concentration and memory, sleep and mood disturbances, headaches, and frequent sore throats and swollen glands. Generally the physical examination and laboratory tests give normal results. Like fibromyalgia, CFS must be diagnosed by looking at signs and symptoms while ruling out disorders that mimic CFS.

Laboratory testing does not contribute to CFS diagnosis except to exclude other conditions (Table 3). Nevertheless, some physicians and patients refuse to recognize CFS without laboratory evidence of abnormal immune function or antibody response to specific infectious agents. They insist that CFS must have infectious or immunologic roots. This idea seems logical, and its continuing pursuit by researchers may yet bear fruit. But so far, extensive studies have failed to link any infectious agent with most cases of CFS. Antibodies to viruses such as human herpesvirus 6 have been found in patients with CFS (40). However, while antibodies are proof of prior infection, they are not proof that the agent of infection caused CFS. Their presence might just as well (and more likely) show that the infectious process, as in a viral infection or Lyme disease, somehow *triggered* CFS (43,44).

Likewise, we know that chronic infections can cause immune disturbances (even after the infection has passed), so antibodies might be evidence of immune alterations that could cause CFS. But, again, extensive studies have found nothing conclusive. Some modest immune alterations have been found in patients with CFS, but such findings are present in many chronic illnesses. Evidence has not been found linking CFS with profound immune abnormalities, yet some people label it "chronic fatigue *immune dysfunction* syndrome."

As with fibromyalgia, CFS research has returned to examine the role of the nervous system, but with a new focus: the interaction of neurohormones with the immune system. The neurologic disturbances, mood disturbances, and sleep disturbances of CFS might best be explained by changes in the central nervous system. Magnetic resonace imaging (MRI) and single photon emission computed tomography (SPECT) scans have revealed alterations of brain blood perfusion in CFS, as well as in fibromyalgia (45). Neuroendocrine studies have found abnormalities in the hypothalamic-pituitary-adrenal axis (46). Some CFS patients have been shown to have neurally mediated hypotension (fall in blood pressure) during the tilt-table test (47).

So progress continues and, as in fibromyalgia, research suggests that CFS is not caused by a single infectious agent, immune alteration, or any other one factor. Instead, it is a complicated illness usually caused by many factors.

Unfortunately, the back and forth declarations that CFS is an infectious disease, an immune disease, or a neurohormonal disorder have not been helpful. They have only added to the dilemma and uncertainty of patients and physicians trying to care for them. These rigid positions have also turned certain CFS support groups against investigators who are miscast as traitors (48). These are researchers whose initial studies suggested that CFS was caused by infection or immune problems, but whose later studies have not borne this out. They are now suspected of concluding that CFS is "all in the mind."

The support groups are understandably sensitive to such a conclusion, but unfair in their suspicion. Most of the "traitors" believe mind and body to be *interrelated* in causing CFS, as discussed in Chapter 12. Modern medicine is moving away from past tendencies to separate mind and body, to attribute a given disorder to one or the other. The mind vs. body approach has been deleterious for people with both fibromyalgia and CFS, as shown by the following case history.

Anna: Fibromyalgia and chronic fatigue syndromes

Anna is a 37-year-old female who told me she had felt exhausted for much of the previous four years. Her illness began with a severe flu, and after that she had never felt well. Anna also complained of muscle aches and extreme sensitivity when her muscles and skin were touched. The fatigue was the most overwhelming symptom, and interfered with much of her daily life. She woke up feeling exhausted and after a few hours of minor activity, she needed a nap. Anna more recently had noted difficulty concentrating. She also began forgetting how to perform simple tasks.

Anna had difficulty getting to sleep, and could not stop her mind from "racing" at night. She was often awakened by her husband's snoring, which would then keep her from getting back to sleep. Anna often did not fall asleep until 4:00 in the morning, and slept best from 6:00 a.m. to 9:00 a.m. She had become quite anxious about these sleep disturbances. Anna told me that she felt very despondent and hopeless in the past year.

Other physicians had told her that she was depressed and very anxious, yet she had never had symptoms of depression or anxiety before all this began, and she had no family history of significant mood disturbances.

The fatigue, disturbed sleep, and muscle aches were continual but became more intense at the time of her menstrual cycle. She had also been getting more viral illnesses, like the flu, and recovery took longer. Her illness had markedly affected her self-esteem, which in the past had been fueled by working long hours in a successful health care marketing position and doing a lot of exercise. Because of her fatigue, she stopped exercising two years ago and had to stop working one year ago.

Various anti-depressants, including Prozac, Zoloft, Wellbutrin, Trazodone, and Effexor had been prescribed. She found herself to be acutely sensitive to very small amounts. Side-effects such as dizziness or agitation prevented her from staying on them for more than a few weeks. Most recently, she had been tolerating 10 mg. of Prozac in the morning. In the past few months it had definitely made her feel better, particularly in the way she was coping with her illness. However, she had recently stopped taking the Prozac and felt increased fatigue and pain. Her doctors had referred her to a Pain Management Center, where nerve blocks (injections of an anesthetic and corticosteroids) did not decrease the pain. However, she did find that modest exercise, heat, or baths gave her short-term pain relief. Ibuprofen, such as six to eight Advil a day, was also helpful for her pain. She had taken Ambien on an as-needed basis, which helped her sleep. Also, Tylenol at night time had been helpful. She was concerned about becoming addicted to needing medications to get to sleep.

Anna's most distressful pain was in the muscles of the neck, shoulders, back, and chest wall. She had cold sensitivity and Raynaud's phenomenon. Anna mentioned that "even my scalp aches." Her laboratory tests included a normal complete blood count (CBC), a normal erythrocyte sedimentation rate (ESR),

and normal immunologic tests for lupus (SLE) or other con-
nective tissue disease. She also had normal thyroid function
tests and a normal chemistry profile. On physical examination,
the patient looked healthy. She had a normal examination other
than the finding of numerous very tender muscles and tendons
in locations that are typically painful in the fibromyalgia syn-
drome.

This case history is typical of someone with either CFS
or fibromyalgia. In general, I no longer separate the two
diagnoses because the symptoms and course of the two
illnesses are so similar (Table 6). I explained this to Anna,
noting that fibromyalgia and CFS may be essentially the
same disorder, just seen from different viewpoints by both
patients and the medical profession. We talked about the
evidence that various stressors, including a viral infection,
can trigger these poorly understood syndromes. I explained why antibiotics or antiviral agents were not likely
to help.

Once Anna understood that she was unlikely to find
the exact cause or cure of her illness, she began to focus
on feeling better. She found it very helpful that her husband had come to our discussion session, since she felt
that he had not been too supportive of her situation. He
admitted that after all the years of her symptoms and the
fact that "she always looked healthy and her tests were
normal," he had begun to question the reality of her complaints. During the next year, their relationship improved.
They began to do much more together as a couple and
were much happier.

Anna was restarted on a low dose of Prozac, 10 mg
taken each morning. Within three weeks she noted improvement in her energy. She also began to sleep better
and started to do regular water exercise and a muscle
stretching routine. She joined a support group run by our
clinical nurse specialist and gradually found that she was

able to do more activities with less pain and less fatigue. When I saw her recently she was doing very well, was back to working full-time, and felt much happier.

At present, there is no highly effective treatment for CFS. My own treatment program for this syndrome is essentially the same as for fibromyalgia (Table 7). We educate people about their illness and how to cope with it. We discuss ways to conserve energy, but also suggest modest regimens for muscle stretching and cardiovascular activity. I often prescribe the same medications that are helpful in fibromyalgia. As detailed in Chapter 14, the fatigue often improves with a serotonin reuptake inhibitor drug. Sleep disturbances are treated with selective medications. If patients feel faint or dizzy when getting up from a chair or out of bed, they may have postural hypotension. If tilt-table testing then demonstrates a neurally mediated hypotension, I will ask the patient to liberalize their salt intake. I may also treat them with medication to increase their blood pressure and pulse response. This treatment alleviates fatigue for some people.

The questionable theory that infections or immune dysfunction cause CFS has led to scientific studies of a variety of treatments including acyclovir, an antiviral agent directed at the EBV virus, and intravenous gammaglobulin to shore up the immune system. These studies, in which subjects receiving treatment were compared with controls (subjects not receiving treatment) found neither to be effective in a reproducible or consistent way. Other controlled studies have shown no significant benefit from injectable liver extract, essential fatty acids, or magnesium.

Despite such negative results, most CFS patients come to me having tried numerous dietary supplements, herbal and "natural" approaches, and certain "immunologic" therapies (see Chapter 10,16). These alternative therapies are often purported to cure people or make them feel better. If they truly do, clinicians must prove it by running controlled studies and publishing the results for the medical community. It is not enough to have subjects try a treatment and give positive testimony. The fact is that people with any disorder often "feel better," at least in the short term, just because they are taking something that is supposed to help. This has been scientifically proven by giving people dummy treatment, or *placebo*, and comparing them to matched controls who receive no dummy pills. Those receiving the dummy pills often improve: the placebo effect. (In Latin, *placebo* means "I will please.")

As might be expected, patients with CFS and/or fibromyalgia share a similar prognosis, or outlook for the future. Generally, those followed in a tertiary referral setting don't do as well as those seen in a primary care or community setting. As explained in the last chapter, most patients receiving tertiary care have been referred to a specialist by a generalist who has been unable to help them. They tend to have a longer history of symptoms or a more complicated problem. They are certainly more discouraged, frustrated, and perhaps even angry because doctors have not helped and have sometimes "not believed them."

In one university specialty referral setting, only 2 percent of CFS patients reported a complete resolution of all of their symptoms an average of 1.5 years after initial evaluation (49). However, most patients do improve, especially those seen in a community setting. In both fibromyalgia and CFS, physician reassurance and a positive outlook go a long way in managing these poorly understood disorders.

SECTION II:
ASSOCIATED CHRONIC ILLNESSES

Chapter 4:
Back pain

I n 1980, I began to have progressively severe low back pain. At the time I was an associate professor at a Boston medical school, balancing patient care, teaching, research, writing, and administrative responsibilities. Intermittent, mild back pain had begun about three years before, but nothing turned up on examination. It bothered me only a little so I ignored it. However, when suddenly it was much worse—present most of every day—I was admitted to the university hospital where I worked.

The neurosurgeon who took care of me suspected a herniated disc in my lower back. He planned surgery, to be preceded by a myelogram (this was in the days before CAT scans and MRIs). This study showed a complete obstruction of the spinal canal in my lower back, which is unusual in cases of herniated discs. However, the next day I had the back surgery (a laminectomy). For the next few days I was too doped up to wonder what had caused the spinal obstruction.

It turned out that the tissue removed from my back was a tumor, not a herniated disc. Naturally I feared it was malignant. Waiting five days for the final pathology report seemed like an eternity. Fortunately, the tumor was benign. No radiation or chemotherapy would be necessary, and recurrence was extremely remote. Patty and I were overcome with relief. But I'll never forget those five dark days of uncertainty and despair over my health and future. Nor will I forget that experience with chronic pain.

At some time in life, one third of Americans have a chronic pain problem. The three most common are chronic back pain, chronic headaches, and fibromyalgia (Table 2). More than 50 million Americans are partially or totally disabled by a chronic pain problem, which costs the country 60-80 billion dollars per year in lost productivity and medical costs (50). At any given time, back pain plagues 80 percent of Americans, costing the nation $14 billion per year (50,51).

Yet little medical interest or research has focused on understanding such disorders. Surprisingly, most medical students receive no formal training in dealing with chronic pain! Nor is there a consistent approach to treatment. In this age of medical subspecialization, each discipline treats pain differently. Internists use drugs, orthopedists remove "slipped" discs, anesthesiologists try nerve blocks, neurosurgeons cut pain pathways, and psychiatrists explore emotional or stress-related causes. Historically, medicine has tried to overlook pain, considering it a "normal" part of healing. It seems that the more sophisticated our biotechnology, the more we neglect chronic pain.

In contrast, acute pain has been well studied. We understand its pathology and its function. When you touch a hot stove, you need not think about making a conscious response. The nerve receptors in your fingers relay a message to your brain, which triggers instantaneous withdrawal. You may think that you pull away from a stove because it hurts but actually, your body engineers this reaction to minimize tissue destruction. Acute pain spreads from our sensory nerves to the central nervous system in a precise and reproducible pathway. The duration of pain corresponds to the duration and nature of the painful stimulus.

Chronic pain seldom follows typical neural pathways. It persists long after the natural and expected response to a stressful stimulus. In fact, it often persists after the initial trauma has healed. Days or weeks after an injury or inflammation, we see no localized pathology—yet our brains do not turn off the pain message. Clearly, chronic pain is a complex process that involves thought, behavior, mood, and motivation. But its exact cause is not at all clear. Eventually, the pain takes on a life of its own that is full of uncertainty.

A striking example is "phantom limb pain." This pain associated with a lost limb is experienced by 50-80 percent of amputees. They describe sensations of burning and tingling and, most strange, actual "presence" or movement where the limb was. These sensations generally fade in a month or two after amputation but can last for years. (Interestingly, studies show that phantom limb pain is more likely to occur and persist if, before amputation, the patient had chronic pain in that limb.) Certainly this phenomenon is a dramatic example of faulty brain-body interaction resulting in pain that cannot be explained by structural or physiologic abnormalities.

Back pain is the most common cause of work loss in the United States. Fortunately, most of it is acute and disappears within a few days or weeks. Acute back pain is usually caused by a muscle "pull" or other tissue injury that responds well to rest, gentle stretches, and simple analgesics like aspirin. However, recurrent or chronic back pain is a major health issue. It is the chief complaint of more than half of all disabled workers who receive compensation.

In 90 percent of people with chronic back pain, the exact cause is uncertain (51). Of course, the examining physician must rule out treatable causes such as herniated disc, spinal stenosis, osteoporosis and vertebral fractures, or tumors of the spine. But all these are rare, so an extensive (and expensive) diagnostic search for the cause is often an unrewarding wild-goose chase.

Both patients and physicians can easily get carried away by our great advances in biotechnology. For example, some patients with chronic back pain insist that I order expensive magnetic resonance imaging of their back. However, MRI detects a disc or joint "abnormality" (simply from normal wear and tear) in half of all people past middle age. Many of them have no back pain at all (52). The MRI often shows some incidental disc protrusion (misnamed "slipped discs") which, again, has nothing to do with chronic back pain. Patients with such protrusions who have surgery to cure their back pain will be very disappointed. The 1960s and 1970s saw a large number of failed back operations in the United States because of the misguided notion that surgery was a panacea for many types of back pain.

Fortunately, indications for surgery on the spine are now much better defined. "Disc" surgery is usually restricted to patients with unremitting pain that has failed non-surgical treatment and who have neurologic impairment. But, most chronic back pain remains frustrating for both the patient and treating physicians, as shown below.

Patient J.T.: Chronic back pain

Jonathan is a 34-year-old mechanic who first experienced back pain at work in 1984, when handling heavy machinery and doing a lot of lifting. He took 3 months off from work and the pain improved. However, when back at work, he fell on some loose tiles and his back pain worsened. The pain was confined to his lower back, with a constant, dull ache that was aggravated by standing and sitting, and improved with lying down. X-ray results were normal, but an MRI done 6 months later demonstrated lumbar disc protrusion. Over the next year, he saw three different surgeons. Two recommended spinal surgery, and one neurosurgeon suggested a course of physical therapy. He cautioned Jonathan to avoid surgery since there were no neurologic abnormalities.

In 1986, Jonathan underwent the first of three back operations. After the first, he felt less pain for about 6 months, but then the pain returned. A second procedure to remove scar tissue was performed in 1988; eventually he had a lumbar spinal fusion in 1990. None of these procedures helped his pain. When I first met Jonathan, he was in constant pain and very limited in his activities. Although he hated taking pain medications, he was continuously using narcotic pain relievers to get through the day. He had to lie down every few hours. His wife worked full-time to support the family. In 1989, Jonathan was declared permanently disabled by the social security disability agency. He received workers' compensation and then spent the next five years in an unresolved law suit against his former employer.

Jonathan told me that he felt hopeless and useless. He never slept for more than a few hours in a row, and could not fall asleep until 1 or 2 a.m. He felt angry at the medical profession for "messing up my back forever." He was most frustrated with physicians who "did not believe him."

Jonathan talked slowly and with a sense of despair. His examination demonstrated no significant neurologic abnormalities. He was very stiff, and the slightest movement of his neck, back, or hips caused severe pain.

This scenario is all too common. Most chronic back pain is not caused by any structural bone or joint abnormalities. It cannot be cured with surgery. Back surgery should be strictly reserved for patients with significant nerve compression who have unremitting symptoms that fail to respond to non-surgical measures. Initial treatment for back pain should include physical therapy, stretching and strengthening back exercises, pain medications, and muscle relaxants (Table 8).

Many types of physical therapy can help patients with chronic back pain. All seek to increase mobility and motion, in stark contrast to treatment of back pain over most of the past 50 years. During that time, the theory was that the back was injured, so it should be rested. Movement was to be avoided. Patients with back pain were often treated with prolonged bed rest, forced inactivity, back braces, or back traction. Physicians now recognize that the longer back motion is restricted, the more difficult it is to rehabilitate the back. For people who grew up under the old approach, this new concept is sometimes difficult to grasp or accept.

Treatment of any chronic pain should above all promote patient independence. For example, Jonathan had been treated by a chiropractor twice a week for four years. This initially helped, then hit a plateau for which the chiropractor recommended frequent "adjustments" to keep the spine in alignment. Chiropractic treatment can help back pain, especially when the pain is acute. However, no treatment for chronic pain should be indefinitely continued unless clear-cut improvement is seen.

Besides his pain, Jonathan was also suffering from depression, sleep disturbances, and a great loss of self-esteem. I started him on medications to treat his depression and to treat his sleep disturbances. He then started a daily water exercise program and physical therapy. Gradually, he noted lessening of his pain as well as improvement in his overall well-being and self-esteem.

However, Jonathan was distressed by the ongoing litigation. He felt that someone was always watching him— that physicians and his insurance company believed he was exaggerating his pain to avoid working. Yet he said he was desperate to return to go back to work. Once litigation was finally resolved, he felt "like a weight has been lifted." After two years of counseling and gradually increased physical therapy, he began a vocational rehabilitation program. When I last saw him, he was working part-time, swimming daily, and had stopped taking narcotic analgesics.

Chapter 5:
Insomnia

I have often had trouble sleeping, even as a child. About four years ago, the problem became much more frequent and I almost never slept well. My mind was always "racing" at bedtime. Usually I would worry about what needed to be done at work; then I would worry about how I'd get it done without sufficient sleep! I became obsessed with sleep and tried counting sheep and other methods. After reading books about relaxation methods (53,54), I tried the "body scan," relaxing myself from head to toe— but with little success. I've never enjoyed drinking but tried, on a few occasions, to lull myself to sleep with a glass of wine or brandy. That would put me to sleep for a few hours, but then I'd be wide awake again.

Eventually, I began to take sleeping medications or "tranquilizers" like Klonopin. Although this medication helped me to sleep, I would often wake at 4 or 5 a.m. Often I felt hung over the next day. Then I began to wake up frequently during the few hours of sleep that I was getting. Finally, I had periods of no sleep, including one lasting three days.

After awhile I hated going to bed. I became short-tempered and resentful of the fact that my wife could fall asleep easily. She would sometimes make snoring noises, which I blamed for my trouble falling asleep. Things got out of hand one night when I was lying awake at 2 a.m., seething, as Patty innocently snored next to me. I actually woke her up and yelled that she was keeping me awake. We had a major argument and she left the room in tears. I felt terrible.

One hundred million Americans have intermittent sleep problems (55). One in six of us has chronic insomnia that interferes with daily life. However, most sleep problems do not have a structural cause; they are not due to a brain or cardiac or respiratory abnormality.

Both normal and abnormal sleep are understood much better than ten years ago because of work in sleep laboratories (55,56). We now know that normal sleep consists of two major phases. Rapid eye movement (REM) sleep, which is when we dream, normally makes up 10-30 percent of sleeping time. The rest is non-REM sleep, which varies from light to deep in four stages. The most important for restoring our energy is stage 4 non-REM sleep—the deepest—which normally makes up 20-30 percent of total sleeping time.

What causes these many phases and stages? Sleep is a complicated process regulated by brain chemicals centered in the hypothalamus, a crucial part of the brain. These chemicals, or neurohormones, transmit electrical impulses throughout the central and peripheral nervous system. Sleep is also regulated by an internal biologic clock. Like all animals, we have a rest-activity cycle, or circadian rhythm. In humans it happens to be about 24 hours, regardless of efforts to change our schedule.

Sleep has important chemical physiologic effects (57,58). We enter stage 4 non-REM sleep with peak concentrations of growth hormone but low levels of cortisol, the "stress hormone." Our body temperature, pulse rate, and breathing rate all are lowered during this stage. Stage 4 seems to be crucial to recovery from the stress of daily life. It is also important to our immune system because a potent immune modulator, interleukin, is largely secreted during this stage (59). Sleep abnormalities that deprive us of Stage 4 non-REM sleep can therefore interfere with our immune function. We may be less able to combat infections and other trauma.

Specific sleep disturbances have characteristic brain wave patterns that can be recorded by electroencephalogram (EEG) in a sleep laboratory. Typically, many small painless sensors are attached to subjects whose brain wave activity and respiration are then monitored as they sleep overnight or for some other period. Though the sensors are often mistakenly associated with electrodes and "shock treatment," they simply read and record impulses.

Sleep EEG studies are the best way to detect obstructive sleep apnea, one of the few structural causes of sleep loss (60,61). People with this condition wake many times in the night because they briefly stop breathing. Their loss of air (*a-pnea*) is brief so that they are rarely in danger. Their waking and resulting sleep loss are so minimal that they often don't notice the problem, especially if they sleep alone. However, they may snore heavily and wake frequently to gasp for air, which can be frightening. The condition is much more common than we used to think, affecting 2-4 percent of adults (61). Most are never properly diagnosed.

People with sleep apnea—or those who sleep near them—will eventually feel sleepy during the day because of sleep loss. Often associated with abnormal cardiopulmonary function (60), sleep apnea should be considered and ruled out by physicians treating anyone who complains of sleep loss. Its causes are often mysterious. Obesity may play a role in the obstruction, but many people with sleep apnea are not particularly overweight. Other causes of airway obstruction, like a very short neck or severe sinus problems, may be involved. In any case, it can often be alleviated by reducing the cause of upper airway resistance. Patients usually do this by wearing a positive-pressure breathing mask at night.

For most people who have trouble falling asleep or staying asleep, the problem is not sleep apnea. Instead, they usually are deficient in their stage 4 non-REM sleep and in their total sleep period (55). Some fall asleep quite easily, then suffer many wakeful periods during the night. Even if they extend their sleep time to counter this loss, they do not feel refreshed in the morning. This "non-restorative sleep" is the most common sleep disturbance reported by people with fibromyalgia and chronic fatigue (62).

Quite a different sleep pattern is more typical of clinical depression. Most depressed patients have a very long sleep latency, that is, the time required to fall into deep sleep (55,56). They sometimes appear to have lost alignment with their circadian rhythm. In fact, depression sometimes improves with "realignment" by deliberate sleep deprivation.

Another pattern of sleep disturbance is seen with *restless leg syndrome* (63). More formally called nocturnal myoclonus, this syndrome involves involuntary movements of the arms or legs plus unpleasant, deep sensations of numbness, tingling, and burning. People often describe feelings of creeping, crawling, or aching in their legs, especially the calves. Still other patterns of sleep disturbance can occur with diseases like hypothyroidism and rheumatoid arthritis.

Clearly, it is important that sleep problems should be specifically identified since different patterns require different treatments (55). For example, medications are relatively useless in sleep apnea; whereas, for true insomnia, traditional sleeping pills are often helpful. Of course, patients should usually avoid prolonged use that can lead to temporary "rebound insomnia" when they try later to stop the drugs (55). Most sleeping pills are in the chemical class of benzodiazepines (55). They include clonazepam (Klonopin), lorazepam (Ativan), flurazepam (Dalmane), temazepam (Restoril), and triazolam (Halcion) (Tables 8 and 9). Recent studies demonstrate that these medications are very safe and rarely addicting (64,65).

Low doses of the tricyclic antidepressants, such as amitriptyline (Elavil), have restored deep sleep for many patients with fibromyalgia and CFS (Table 9). These medications seem to push people into deeper sleep, and can also decrease pain and relax muscles. If muscle and joint pain cause wakefulness, acetaminophen or non-steroidal anti-inflammatory medications (NSAIDs) can be taken at bedtime (Table 8).

Insomnia is rarely a sign of a specific disease but is quite commonly related to a chronic illness or to stress. Like chronic pain and chronic fatigue, insomnia can point to physical and emotional upheaval. Therefore, treatment must focus on multiple factors, beginning with some non-medicinal steps. Insomnia combined with mood disturbances will often improve if those disturbances are addressed with counseling. Also, patients can learn better sleep habits. They can attend behavioral-modification programs now offered at many hospitals (66) or work on their own. Either way, they need to know the following basic sleep facts and guidelines.

Individuals vary greatly in the sleep they need. Some people truly need the traditional 8 hours per night, but many do very well on 5-7. In general, most of us think we need more sleep than we actually do. Sleep research has found that humans can be totally deprived of sleep for 7-10 days with remarkably little effect on their physical or mental abilities (55). The right amount of sleep for you involves no tricky formulas. It is simply the amount that makes you feel most alert. That amount tends to decrease for adults as they age, so we will awake more easily and often as we get older.

Caffeine, smoking, and alcohol interfere with sleep. If your spouse snores or the room is noisy, try ear plugs or a generator of "white noise." Keep the room cool. Avoid heavy meals late in the evening. Regular exercise will help sleep, but should be avoided near bedtime since it causes temporary stimulation.

When you have trouble getting to sleep, it usually means that you are anxious about something—or you are simply not ready to go to sleep. Experiment with less sleep by going to bed later than usual, then getting up at your accustomed time. In general, if you lie awake more than 30 minutes, it is best to get up. Read or do something else relaxing until you feel sleepy. Don't lie there tossing and turning and getting frustrated, as I did for years! Another bad habit of mine, which many people share, is looking repeatedly at the clock when lying awake. I finally turned it around so it couldn't distract me, but could still wake me in the morning. Relaxation techniques of any type can help you fall asleep. If you have pain in your muscles and joints, take some aspirin or acetaminopen or ibuprofen at bedtime.

Most important, do not obsess about lack of sleep. This will not help you relax! Trust your body to readjust itself and get the sleep it needs, sooner or later. Most sleep problems tend to go away as mysteriously as they came on. Soon you'll return to your old sleeping habits. Meanwhile, your sleep loss may not cause the problems you fear. During the height of my insomnia and depression, I had to give an important lecture to physicians affiliated with Harvard medical school. I was apprehensive about it and couldn't concentrate to arrange my slides and practice the night before. I had no sleep at all that night, and next day gave the lecture feeling sleepy and ill-prepared.

Yet apparently the lecture did not suffer because it went without a hitch and generated many good comments from my colleagues.

We all need our sleep. But we probably need less than we think. Worrying too much about it will only add to your sleep woes.

Chapter 6:
Irritable Bowel Syndrome

Most patients with fibromyalgia and CFS also have irritable bowel syndrome (IBS). As with each of the illnesses described in this book, this is diagnosed by specific criteria. They include a change in bowel habits, usually with alternating diarrhea and constipation and abdominal pain (67). There is often abdominal distention, or bloating; cramping and subsequent pain relief with bowel movements; mucus in the stool, and the sensation of incomplete evacuation.

As with the pain of fibromyalgia, these symptoms are most likely to represent IBS if they have persisted at least three months. Meanwhile, the physician must rule out diseases having similar symptoms, especially since they may lend themselves to specific treatment. Such diseases include gastritis or peptic ulcer disease and inflammatory bowel diseases, such as ulcerative colitis or Crohn's colitis. They must be ruled out by a careful history and physical examination, as well as certain tests. These usually include sigmoidoscopy or colonoscopy and radiologic examination of the bowel.

At some time in their lives, 10-20 percent of Americans suffer IBS-like symptoms. The symptoms are so common as to account for 25-50 percent of all visits to a gastroenterologist. However, since symptoms often suggest ordinary indigestion, many people never seek medical attention. According to some estimates, half the people in the community who have these symptoms are never actually diagnosed or treated (67).

Irritable bowel syndrome is three times more common in women than in men (67,68). Its cause and development are very similar to that of the other chronic illnesses that we are discussing. They are each currently thought to involve an interplay of physical and psychosocial factors. The physical factors in IBS include altered bowel motility because of a disturbance in peristalsis. This is the automatic wave-like mechanism by which the bowel wall pushes waste products through the intestines. For some reasons as yet unknown, peristalsis can hit a snag. It fails to operate smoothly, causing short-term stoppage, cramping, and bloating. From person to person, episodes vary widely in frequency and severity. They usually begin and end mysteriously.

Another physical factor seen in IBS is that patients have a lower than normal pain threshold in response to gut distention (67). In other words, they feel pain at a level of bloating that would not cause such discomfort in other people.

Studies have shown an increased prevalence of depression, anxiety, and physical abuse or sexual abuse in people with IBS (67). It is important to emphasize, however, that this research focused on people with IBS who went to a gastroenterologist or other specialist (67,68). As far as we know, increased prevalence of such problems is not found in IBS victims not seeing a specialist. In other words, such psychosocial factors as depression and prior abuse may not predict who develops IBS, but only how people will react to their illness: who will seek help, who will deny or play the stoic.

Psychosocial and stress factors are very important in understanding the response to chronic illness from one person to another. Factors may be simple and straightforward, such as current unhappiness at home or work. They may be more complex and hidden, such as childhood abuse of some kind. Our minds can completely bury our most unpleasant experiences. We may gloss over or entirely suppress emotional and physical trauma such as childhood sexual abuse. Therapy that uncovers such abuse has become very controversial because, although many results are genuine, suggestible patients have been prompted by leading questions to imagine such episodes. However, accurate estimates suggest that (shockingly!) 20-30 percent of the general population have suffered at least one episode of such physical or sexual abuse.

Most studies suggest a slightly higher than normal incidence of childhood abuse among adults who suffer irritable bowel syndrome, fibromyalgia and other chronic pain disorders (69-71).

Jane: Irritable bowel syndrome

Jane had a history of gastrointestinal problems beginning at age 5. She always had either constipation or loose bowel movements, often with cramping. Her mother had ulcerative colitis, and Jane was initially diagnosed with that disease. However, extensive studies, including a biopsy of her intestine, finally ruled out inflammatory bowel disease.

Jane was an outstanding student and athlete in high school. She was a superb gymnast and at one point had considered moving to Texas and training to be an Olympic gymnast. During high school, she had few friends and rarely dated. Jane did very well academically at an Ivy League college. However, in her junior year, she lost 15 pounds and her chronic bowel irritability was worse than ever. In order to counter this, she stopped eating many foods and, in retrospect, told me that she had a six-month stretch of bulimia that year. Jane said that in college, it was "fashionable" to make a habit of vomiting after eating.

I met Jane during her senior year at college. She had begun to feel very fatigued and noted abdominal, pelvic, and back pain. She was referred to me to investigate whether arthritis was a factor.

I found no evidence of arthritis. Her physical examination and laboratory tests were completely normal. She was very thin, was 5 feet, 4 inches tall, and weighed 88 pounds. At first she was quiet and withdrawn but as we talked she became more animated. When I asked her about her childhood history of bowel trouble, she began to cry. After a few minutes of silence, she told me that her bowel problems began at a time when she was verbally and physically abused by her stepfather. She had never discussed this with her mother for fear that her mother's ulcerative colitis would become worse.

Jane agreed to see a mental health professional to work out the issues of her childhood trauma. At first, this was very difficult for her. But eventually her emotional state improved, and she became more open and outgoing. With a change in her diet and avoidance of lactose-containing foods, her bowel symptoms also improved. She began to regain weight lost in college and was much less obsessed about her weight and diet.

Jane's physical and mental well-being both needed attention. Education about IBS and its "benign" nature were very reassuring to her. Elimination of certain foods, such as dairy products or legumes, is often helpful in IBS. Adding more fiber to the diet usually makes bowel habits more regular. Antidiarrheal or anticonstipation medications can be used, depending on which symptoms predominate. When pain, gas, and bloating occur, they may be alleviated by antispasmodic agents such as belladonna or dicyclomine.

Interestingly, tricyclic antidepressants, as used in fibromyalgia, CFS, low back pain, and migraine, are often useful to treat the abdominal pain and cramps associated with IBS (67). Whether these medications work as antidepressants, anticholinergics, or analgesics is unclear.

Non-medicinal therapies used in IBS have included biofeedback, hypnotherapy, and psychotherapy. Acceptance of the uncertain diagnosis and treatment is an important step, as with the other syndromes discussed. Early diagnosis and minimal use of invasive testing will help alleviate discomfort, fear, and anxiety for people suffering from this common disorder.

Chapter 7:
Migraine and Other Headaches

Last year I began to experience headaches that were more severe than any I'd had before. They were paroxysmal, or intermittent, and occurred primarily on one side of my head, around my eye and temple. Hippocrates and his ancient colleagues puzzled over such headaches of the *hemicranion* or "half-cranium." Over the next 2500 years, the Greek word lost its head and tail to become the French word *migraine*. However, all those centuries did not reveal a cause or cure.

My headaches were "classic" migraines that began with a visual aura of shimmering light waves and lines. Sometimes I saw strange objects and geometric shapes or movement, almost like blips across a radar screen (72). When the aura began, I knew the headache was about to explode. Often it brought transient nausea or sensations of numbness and tingling to my face or one arm. It might bring nasal stuffiness and watery eyes, making me wonder whether to blame the headache on my old allergies and sinus problems. I became very sensitive to light and noise.

The headaches would usually disappear in a few hours, especially if I took a lot of aspirin. What helped me most was to lie down in a dark room, perfectly still. If I could fall asleep, I usually awoke without the headache. However, a severe episode would leave several hours of exhaustion in its wake.

These headaches became more frequent and then lost their aura. This made them no longer "classic" but "common migraine", but the pain did not feel common to me! Sometimes the headaches became nearly continuous—a migraine storm—and interfered with my work and sleep. I spent hours trying to figure out what I was doing wrong. I tinkered with my diet and wondered if I was getting too much or too little sleep. Was I doing too much exercise? Could the headaches be caused by fumes I was breathing somewhere? Naturally I considered they might be caused by work-related stress, since at first they only occurred at work. But later they ambushed me on weekends too.

Preoccupied and looking for a diagnosis, I saw my internist, an ear-nose-and throat specialist, an allergist, an opthalmologist, and a neurologist. I tried pain medications, muscle relaxants, anti-inflammatory medications, and medications that specifically treat migraine (see Chapter 14). The neurologist tried Midrin, a commonly prescribed analgesic (pain reliever) for migraine. He also put me on a beta-blocker, propanolol, to help prevent the migraine attacks—a common strategy. Then he tried Imitrex, which can help to knock out acute attacks of migraine. None of these medicines helped much.

At this point I compounded the problem with two mistakes that I now warn my patients against. First, I began to orchestrate my own care and consultations. Second, I sought advice from too many sources. Of course, these traps are more likely to snare health care professionals when they become ill. They are surrounded by resources and have many colleagues with whom to exchange information and services free of charge.

Each year in the United States there are 18 million visits to the doctor for evaluation and treatment of headaches

(73). In fact, headaches are the most common symptom that bring people to see a physician. As with syndromes like fibromyalgia and CFS, the exact causes of most headaches are not understood. Very occasionally, they may be an early sign of a serious underlying illness such as cancer, stroke, or infection. However, the vast majority do not signal disease, nor do they stem from any brain or skull problem. They can be divided roughly into two main groups: muscular or "tension" headaches and vascular or migraine headaches.

Muscular headaches are typically associated with spasm and tenderness in the neck, face, and shoulder muscles. They are usually persistent; that is, they last for days or weeks at a time. People report that the pain feels like "a band constricting around my head." It is often aggravated by turning the head or looking up. Many people describe pain and numbness in the face and jaw. The muscles of the head, neck, and face are often very tender when touched.

For lack of a better diagnosis, most patients with these chronic headaches and neck, facial, or jaw pain are told they have "tension headaches." This implies that their pain is a manifestation of "psychic tension," but no solid research supports this theory. There is no evidence that people with these headaches have more psychic stress or tension than other people. The truth is that the cause of these headaches is unknown. However, muscular headaches may sometimes be caused by structural problems of the jaw, teeth, or neck.

Temporomandibular joint syndrome (TMJ) is often diagnosed when headaches seem related to a malalignment of the jaw. However, as in the next case, the term TMJ is often used loosely or even mistakenly.

Scott: TMJ Syndrome

Scott began complaining of jaw and ear pain following root canal surgery four years ago. Over a 10-month period, he began to get frequent right-sided headaches associated with pain over the right ear, face, neck, and upper back. During the next year, he consulted with a number of dentists, oral surgeons, and two neurologists. He was referred to a dental school maxillo-facial clinic that specialized in TMJ. Extensive X-rays and examinations revealed clicking and some malalignment of the right jaw. Scott was treated with anti-inflammatory medicine, gentle jaw exercises, and neck physical therapy. At night he wore a mouth guard to prevent grinding of the teeth. He improved slightly but still had persistent jaw pain and headaches. He sought another opinion and was told that surgery was necessary. Three years ago he underwent jaw reconstructive surgery.

Unfortunately, after surgery his headaches worsened. He had to wear a mouth splint for three months afterward, which he felt aggravated his headaches and made it difficult to eat. For the next two years, Scott had daily severe headaches to the point that he stopped working. He needed to take frequent naps because of fatigue and he became discouraged and depressed.

Last year, an attorney told him that he should sue the dentist who performed the initial root canal surgery because of medical malpractice. During the 6 months before I saw Scott, he had been engrossed in that malpractice suit. His lawyer had suggested he see me. Upon examination, I found exquisite muscle tenderness and spasm in the right facial, neck, and upper back muscles. The rest of the examination was unremarkable. He stated that he was bitter about the jaw surgery that had made things worse.

I told Scott that he had a localized form of fibromyalgia, termed myofascial pain syndrome (see chapter 2). I discussed how muscles and soft tissues react to chronic pain and explained that, in most instances, surgery will not cure the body's maladaptive reaction. I suggested a return to conservative treatment with medicine and physical therapy. I attempted to convince

Scott while the root canal surgery may have aggravated his
pain, it was not malpractice. I doubt that our discussion changed
his mind since I never heard from Scott or his lawyer again.

Migraine headaches are described as "vascular" because of their throbbing, pulse-like quality. This suggests
that the blood supply to the head is involved. They are
subdivided into "classic" migraine, with visual phenomena or aura and "common" migraine without aura. The
prevalence of migraine in the United States is estimated
at 18 percent for females and 6 percent for males (74).
Since women outnumber men, this works out to 20 million
women and 10 million men. Nearly half of these millions
experience moderate to severe disability.

Migraine is a perfect example of the mind-body or
psychophysiologic illness. Neurologist Oliver Sacks, who
wrote The Man Who Mistook His Wife for a Hat and
Awakenings (made into a movie), previously wrote a
book called Migraine. He has described the impact of
migraine on both the physical and emotional aspects of
well-being (72). Characteristically, the pain and other
physical symptoms occur first, then are followed by severe fatigue, apathy, withdrawal, and depression. Patients often suffer sensitivity to light and noise: *photophobia*
and phonophobia. Stress, certain foods, the timing of a menstrual cycle and hormone replacement therapy (estrogens) may each play a role in bringing on a migraine.

A precise cause or pathophysiologic explanation for
migraine has been as elusive as for chronic fatigue syndrome and fibromyalgia (5) (Figure 1). Scientists have
found genetic factors. They have also found that a migraine with aura is accompanied by a deficiency of oxygen
to the brain. Oxygen is carried by the blood cells, and we
see a gradually diminished blood supply to the brain hem-
isphere where the headaches are most intense (75). Recent

investigations have focused on possible neurohormone disturbances.

As usual, serotonin is one of the suspects. Its release at the site of the migraine causes constriction of cerebral arteries, which could explain the diminished blood supply. In the laboratory, a drug that alters serotonin concentration can induce headaches and also the generalized muscle pain seen in fibromyalgia (76). Thus migraine definitely has biologic features. Like the other illnesses discussed in this book, it is not just a psychosocial phenomenon. A recent editorial in a medical journal warns physicians that many must "change their views and acknowledge that migraine is a neurobiologic, not a psychogenic, disorder" (75).

Patients that I see have often had migraine and tension headaches for most of their lives. Many, like Martin below, also have fibromyalgia and CFS.

Martin: Headaches and chronic pain

Martin is a 55-year-old man who began to experience severe headaches at age 20. These included both "classic" migraine headaches, which occurred about four times per year, and muscular headaches. The migraine attacks were associated with nausea and vomiting, photophobia, and phonophobia. Martin's headaches generally were preceded by a visual aura of formed lines and bright lights. Usually the headaches were most intense on one side of his head and face, but occasionally they were bilateral. They were incapacitating and usually would last one to two days. Martin had gained some relief with analgesics, such as Fiorinal, and with ergotamines, such as Cafergot, but said the migraines still had to run their course. He described his other headaches as a constant pain in the neck and shoulders, as well as the front and back of the head. They had been getting progressively worse and more frequent during the past year.

More recently, Martin was getting the migraine headaches at least twice a week. They were not responding well to medications. Because of the persistent headaches, he had stopped working as an accountant about 6 months before. He also had stopped exercising. During the prior 4 months, Martin had begun to sleep very poorly. He had already seen two neurologists and had a negative work-up, including a normal MRI of the brain. His physical examination was unremarkable except for muscle tenderness and decreased range of motion in the neck and shoulders.

I began Martin on Imitrex, and during the next 6 months he had only one severe attack of migraine. The muscular headaches were treated with acetaminophen and ibuprofen and he began a physical therapy program. He also began a pain management program that included both biofeedback and progressive muscle relaxation. After 3 months of this program, the daily headaches lessened, he resumed an exercise program, and also began to sleep better. He still had frequent muscular headaches, especially when under stress, but was able to resume his job.

Martin's improvement was related to a combination of factors. Certainly, the development of new, more potent and specific medications for migraine has helped many patients. Also, it was important that Martin recognized that he had two different types of headaches (which often trigger each other), each needing its own treatment. His migraines responded best to Imitrex (sumatriptan), a medication developed specifically to treat migraines by changing serotonin levels in the brain (77). His muscular headaches responded best to analgesics, exercise and physical therapy. Both types of headaches improved with relaxation techniques that included biofeedback, yoga, and meditation.

Like many patients who take these steps, Martin did not eliminate his migraines but lessened their pain and hold on his life. As he gained confidence in his improvement and feeling of control, he was able to get back to a normal work and recreational schedule.

Chapter 8:
Thought and memory disturbances

The saga of my headaches continued, and finally I had my first weekend-long migraine. It began Saturday morning and didn't let up. I could not concentrate on anything. That afternoon, in desperation, I did what patients should never do: I borrowed my wife's medication. Patty had been prescribed Elavil for the sleep disturbances and pain associated with fibromyalgia. She had improved markedly with that medicine, which in much higher doses is used to treat depression (78). However, in people not used to taking it, this type of medication can cause fatigue, despondency, and a "spaced out" feeling. The whole next day, I could barely get out of bed because of these side effects. On top of everything, I recognized for the first time that my fatigue had been joined by a deep sense of depression. I felt sad and hopeless.

On Monday morning, I had an MRI scan of my brain. Unexpectedly, the scan was much more stressful than the several previous CAT scans of my head and sinuses. Not only are you in a darker and more confined space, but you are assailed by what sounds like a jack-hammer in your ear. Then I waited all day for the results. Finally, at 5:00 p.m. the neurologist called and said: "The good news is you don't have a brain tumor. The bad news is there is some type of growth in the bone of your skull. This is surely benign, but I think you should see our neurosurgeon and have it removed."

I hardly slept the night before my surgery. Patty and I arrived at the hospital at 6:00 a.m. since I was scheduled for an 8:00 a.m. operation. Most surgeons are morning people who like to cut when they are the most alert, which is fine with me! I undressed and put on the "johnnie," wondering where that silly name came from and what idiot had designed this foolish gown. Two catheters were placed in my arms, in an artery and a vein. Suddenly I was transformed from person to patient with a rapidity that has always amazed me. Doctor, lawyer, merchant, chief: as soon as you lie down on that examining table or put on that hospital gown, you become dependent, obedient, and vulnerable. You lose not only your belongings and your clothes, but your dignity.

The surgery on my head was delayed for 2 hours because of some "emergency." Like all patients, I wondered indignantly what emergency could be more important than mine! I tried to stay calm lying on the gurney in a cold, brightly lit space next to the operating room. The guy next to me, about 30-years-old and waiting for knee surgery, kept talking and fidgeting about on his gurney. It was too small for him, but his thrashing about seemed less like discomfort than "nervous anticipation." I practiced my newly-acquired skills of deep breathing/relaxation, but to little avail.

The surgery went well. The skull mass turned out to be a bone infection called osteomyelitis, related to my lifelong sinus problems. The sinus problems would require more surgery. But with more antibiotics to prevent infection and steroids to keep my brain from swelling, the headaches disappeared. Unlike most chronic headaches, mine luckily had a structural cause that had been found and removed.

However, when I awoke from surgery, I was still a patient. Lying in the intensive care unit, with tubes and catheters everywhere, I had a seizure that evening. I had two more over the next three days. Minor seizures or convulsions are not uncommon following brain surgery. In fact, 5% of the population will have a seizure at some time in their lives. They can usually be controlled by medication and seldom fit the thrashing and foaming picture that most people have of convulsions. Most are hardly noticeable unless recorded by EEG. I have no recall of my three seizures, although I could tell by the way that my wife and children looked at me that they must have noticed something strange and scary.

While still at the hospital I had two more brain MRIs since my physicians needed to be certain that I was not developing brain swelling or hemorrhage. Again I was trapped in the MRI machine, feeling cramped and claustrophobic. Finally, five days after surgery, I went home from the hospital armed with two different anti-seizure medications, two antibiotics, and steroids.

At home, I did not know what to fret about first! I thought that the scar on my head looked pretty mean. (The surgeon showed me the post-operative MRI of my head, which demonstrated a large prosthesis where one-quarter of my skull bone used to be.) I was concerned about my blood tests, especially the low number of white blood cells, which my colleagues could not explain. Perhaps most upsetting, I felt dizzy and had trouble concentrating, presumably because of the anti-seizure medications. Reading or any serious pursuit was impossible so I started sleeping during the day. This made me lie awake at night.

One of my most disturbing activities was staring down at my pill box, four times each day. During my first week at home, I was taking more than 20 pills daily! In my fuzzy condition I could hardly keep them straight. I quickly learned the importance of having a labeled pill box.

I continued to feel confused, dizzy, and exhausted. My seizures and adverse reactions to the anti-seizure medications had apparently caused "cognitive disturbances." This phrase covers anything that affects thought and memory. It sounds bland, but nothing is so frightening as a problem that involves the brain. The fear of losing our intellect and our memories is very frightening. Still orchestrating my own care, I kept complaining to the neurologist that I was wiped out from the anti-seizure medications, so he kept changing them around. I was unable to concentrate even on a TV program or a light novel. On top of this, I learned that because of possibly recurrent seizures, I could not drive a car for six months. For Patty this was a big inconvenience; for me, it was a big blow to my sense of masculinity and control over life.

My cognitive problems eventually went away, but gave me insight into patients with chronic illness who sometimes have similar problems. The temporary neurocognitive disturbances seen in patients with fibromyalgia and CFS are quite similar to those seen in people recovering from head trauma or injuries. Their cognitive disturbances are rarely serious or lasting, and cannot be linked with a pathologic cause. There is no inflammation of the central nervous system, as in multiple sclerosis. There is no brain atrophy, as in dementia like Alzheimer's disease. However, the very lack of structural pathology causes some physicians to dismiss the problems as imaginary. At the other extreme, against scientific evidence, patients are sometimes told that they suffer serious brain "damage." Witness the alarmist quote from the cover of the book *Osler's Web:* "CFS is an infectious disease that can devastate the immune system, attack the brain, and leave its victims physically and emotionally over-whelmed..." (48). This all sounds more violent and *permanent* than is actually the case.

Research to determine the cause of thought and memory disturbances after trauma is similar to research in fibromyalgia and CFS that we have discussed. Patients also have many similar symptoms, as reported by Susan:

Susan: Pain and cognitive disturbances

Susan, a 56-year-old female, was healthy until she was involved in a motor vehicle accident six years ago. She was driving, wearing her seat belt, and suffered a "whiplash" injury to her neck. She was seen in an emergency room and had a normal examination and normal X-rays of her skull. During the next year, she continued to have pain and stiffness in her neck and shoulders, with muscular-type headaches. Gradually she began having more difficulty concentrating. She complained especially of losing short-term memory and the ability to process information as quickly as usual. For the first time in her life she began getting very dizzy. Sometimes this would occur with headaches but at other times she would "for no reason" feel dizzy. She described the dizziness as a "loss of my equilibrium." Susan also complained of severe fatigue and sensitivity to noise and light.

Her job as a paralegal assistant became more and more difficult. Gradually she also noted a change in her sleep, waking often at 3 or 4 in the morning. She became very irritable with her family and friends.

Susan saw 2 neurologists and had negative studies, including a spinal tap, 2 CAT scans, and 3 MRIs of her head. She saw a psychiatrist who felt that she was mildly depressed but also diagnosed a "post-concussion-like illness." Neuropsychological testing suggested an adult attention deficit disorder. She was started on Ritalin for the attention problem and Zoloft to treat the depression. Gradually, Susan noted less attention problems and less irritability.

Susan's cognitive problems are called post-concussive or cervicoencephalic syndrome (79). As with similar problems seen in patients with fibromyalgia and CFS, the explanation for these symptoms may lie in decreased blood flow to the brain (80,81). In patients like Susan, the flow of blood and delivery of oxygen might be hampered by wounded and healing tissues. In patients with chronic illness, the flow might instead be hampered by the deficiency of a neurohormone like serotonin. In any case, the resulting difficulties appear mainly to interfere with executive skills. These are the attention abilities that allow us to execute the large and small tasks we normally dispatch without a conscious thought. We can lose these attention abilities temporarily through stress, illness, or injury, or more permanently through normal aging. We tend to interpret the problem as memory loss, but actually it represents difficulty taking in and processing information. There is no evidence of significant brain injury or inflammation.

Dizziness following head injury is very common and has a poorly understood organic basis (82). In such cases, as in CFS and fibromyalgia, vestibular tests reveal abnormalities suggestive of central nervous system deficits (83). Both psychiatric and neural-mediated dizziness are often overlooked and difficult to treat. Sometimes they are mistaken for the dizziness caused by inner ear infections. Furthermore, patients are somewhat more susceptible to develop persistent dizziness and impairment if they have past or current mood disorders (84,85). Such disorders by themselves can cause impairment, which complicates diagnosis and treatment.

An intricate interaction of the mind and body has (yet again!) been postulated to contribute to the neuro-cognitive disturbances seen in chronic illnesses and following trauma. As with Susan, improvement often occurs with time. Antidepressants combined with the "stimulants" given to children with attention deficit disorder (ADD) are often helpful. Some patients may need job retraining or instruction in better self-organization. Such organization simply means more systematic attention to detail: more use of a calendar or daybook, more writing down of complicated directions, and so forth.

Patients with cognitive problems after trauma or during chronic illnesses like fibromyalgia and CFS should be reassured that these symptoms reflect no permanent, structural lesions. They and their physicians should be extremely wary of MRI and PET scans that detect subtle "abnormalities" of the brain. A serious concern with these new high-tech brain imaging techniques is that their "abnormal" findings are not truly abnormal. Like the disc problems discussed earlier, they often do not correlate with any serious pathology. They certainly do not require medical or surgical attention.

The structural and biochemical analysis of the central nervous system is an important area of research in fibromyalgia, chronic fatigue syndrome, migraine and depression (80,81). It may hold important clues to these problems, but more controlled studies are needed. In the meantime, physicians or patients should not leap to accept inconclusive research findings as evidence of brain degeneration!

The cognitive disturbances common to chronic pain, chronic fatigue, and mood disturbances are likely to be multifactorial. Physical and chemical alterations in the central nervous system are only part of the problem. Medications to alleviate seizure or mood or sleep disturbances are frequent causes of thought and memory difficulties. The difficulties are made worse by our natural fear of incurable, progressive deterioration of the nervous system. They are made even worse by pain, sleep loss, and depression.

Fortunately, these thought and memory disturbances usually recede over time. If not, they tend to be only modest problems that do not get worse. Patients with a positive attitude can find creative ways around them.

Chapter 9:
Depression

Some weeks after the surgery for osteomyelitis, I went out of state for surgery to correct my sinus infections. The recuperation was uneventful but I was alone, away from home, and missing the birth of Michael, my first grandson. When I finally saw him, back in Boston, he had spent a day in the neonatal intensive care unit. Now he was fine, but he looked very frail to me. Despite Patty's reassurance, I kept dwelling on the idea that something was wrong with him.

My unreasonable fears about Michael's health were undoubtedly driven by fears for my own health. I was anxious to get back to my normal routine, but still feeling exhausted and overwhelmed. After missing weeks of work, I began to worry about our finances. One night, in the car, I imagined we were about to crash. This terrible end almost seemed to offer relief from the gloom that enveloped me. Fortunately, Patty was driving!

I began to suspect I was becoming dangerously depressed. However, I rationalized these symptoms as the natural consequence of my illnesses, surgeries, and health uncertainties of the past year. I ignored them and returned to work, but had trouble concentrating. Feelings of despair, anger and, above all, fear of the unknown began to again keep me from sleeping. Even with medication, I could not fall asleep for hours. At work, every task seemed overwhelming, and one day I simply ground to a halt. If not for my wife, who works in the office, I would not have made it through the day.

At that point I sought out a primary care physician to manage my multiple illnesses. He spent a lot of time talking to me. He took charge, bringing together all the information from my multiple specialists. He set out a plan for me. Finally I was ready to relinquish control of my health care.

My new physician referred me to a psychiatrist. Intellectually I knew this was a good idea, but I was apprehensive. What if he could not get me out of this funk? What if he thought that had I brought it on myself? The psychiatrist started me on Zoloft, an antidepressant, and we began psychotherapy. I initiated this "talking cure" by blurting out my medical history, my fears that I would never be myself again, and my guilt at making my family suffer. Having heard my own patients catastrophize about their illness, I heard myself sounding exactly the same. I kept thinking, "No one knows what I'm going through." Or, "Why can't I be stronger and handle this better?"

The next month was hard, but Patty's strength countered my own fragility. She had always relied on me, perhaps because I had never allowed myself to rely on her. Now she comforted me and listened to my fears, no matter how unrealistic. We became close in a way that we never had before. For the first time, I saw how well my children understood me and my insecurities. I realized that if I got past this period, I might not be the same person—but maybe that was not the end of the world! Patty and I talked about how we would manage even if I could not return to work. She made this terrible possibility seem like something we could handle. It seemed less frightening, almost like an adventure. However, I withdrew at first from almost everyone else, not wanting to see their sadness or pity. Then I realized how much I needed their contact and affection.

The antidepressant medication and twice-weekly talks with the psychiatrist began to help. I don't know which was more effective, but I believe that together they worked better than either alone. My debilitating depression lifted within a month. I could resume full-time work and exercise, and felt much more under control. Despite still being on a number of medications, I felt better and better about myself and my health.

What kind of depression could take such toll and then completely disappear? Such a course suggests the illness of depression—something more serious than the routine "depression" or discouragement of a bad mood or a bad day. Indeed it is an illness. It is termed "clinical depression" to distinguish it from normal depression. It is "clinical" in having specific signs and symptoms that can be detected by a physician (Table 4).

Clinical depression is often divided into major depression and minor depression (86). Some time in their life, 10-20 percent of Americans will have an episode of major depression, similar to what I experienced. For many, such episodes are recurrent. For a few, major depression becomes chronic and never really lifts. Some people appear to be born with it.

Major depression can be chronic but is most often acute. In contrast, minor depression is more often a chronic problem. Also called dysthymia, it is hard to separate from normal "bad moods." The difference may largely be a matter of degree. Instead of having an occasional bad mood, dysthymic people have one after the other. They are often described as "moody" or "pessimistic" people. Their gloom is not as deep or debilitating as major depression, but it is an ongoing and difficult problem.

Major or minor depression takes a huge toll on our health and well being. These two kinds of clinical depression account for more days lost from work than arthritis, diabetes, chronic lung disease, or hypertension. Especially with major depression, people simply have trouble getting on with life. They sometimes have days when they cannot get out of bed or "put one foot in front of the other." If undiagnosed and untreated, their suicide rate is much higher than among the general population (86). This chapter will focus mainly on major depression, though much of it applies in some degree to minor depression or dysthymia.

The illness of depression is hard to describe but very different from feeling blue. It causes a kind of pain that, in my case, was deeper than anything I had experienced. I felt confused, hopeless, and profoundly sad. As with most chronic illness, I could hardly remember being well and feared I would never return to my old self.

Even a great writer has trouble finding the right words to characterize depression. In his short book, <u>Darkness Visible</u>, William Styron writes: "I was feeling in my mind a sensation close to, but indescribably different from, actual pain...That the word 'indescribable' should present itself is not fortuitous, since it has to be emphasized that if pain were readily describable, most of the countless sufferers from this ancient affliction would have been able to confidently depict for their friends and loved ones (even their physicians) some of the actual dimensions of their torment, and perhaps elicit a comprehension that has been generally lacking; such incomprehension has usually been due not to a failure of sympathy but to a basic inability of healthy people to imagine a form of torment so alien to everyday experience. For myself, the pain is most closely connected to drowning or suffocation—but even those images are off the mark" (87).

Fibromyalgia, CFS, and chronic pain are never fatal in themselves, but on rare occasions the commonly associated depression can be fatal. On Friday, August 17, 1996, three reporters from Boston television stations and newspapers phoned me. They wanted my opinion on the latest suicide assisted by Dr. Jack Kevorkian: a Massachusetts woman with fibromyalgia and CFS. Not knowing her or her situation, I was reluctant to comment. However, I stressed that, among 10,000 patients I'd diagnosed with fibromyalgia and CFS over 18 years, only two had much later taken their lives. I urged the reporters to convey these numbers to the public to demonstrate how very rare suicide is in illnesses like fibromyalgia. It occurs only when such illnesses are accompanied by *untreated* major depression.

The fact that major depression is hard to describe and not visible or clearly "physical" places a whole layer of obstacles in the path of recovery. First of all, people cannot fathom how depression and our reaction to stress could relate to the myriad of bodily symptoms in fibromyalgia and CFS. Even many physicians have trouble with this idea. Yet studies definitely show that mood disturbances generate a whole set of physical symptoms, including abdominal pain, muscle pain, and headaches (88).

Secondly, any suggestion that a person's problems are "mental" instead of "physical" may be seen as a character flaw. Even medically sophisticated people share the Victorian notion that mental illness is a sign of frailty—something to be hidden, from guilt and shame. I myself felt some embarrassment about going to a psychiatrist. What if a colleague or patient saw me? If I arrived early for an appointment, I would wait in my car rather than in his waiting room. Intellectually I knew that visits with a psychiatrist should be no different than visits with any other physician. So why was I hiding in my car?

Of course, there was one good reason. The medically sophisticated person knows that, however enlightened his or her own view of depression and psychiatry, many people will not understand. Our society's continuing failure to accept mood disturbances as "legitimate" illness forces patients to feel embarrassed. It often causes them to deny their depression and avoid treatment that could help them. They must bear loss of self-esteem, along with their depression. They feel frail or inadequate, as I did, and guilty for "bringing this on myself." I now believe that my recurrent bouts of fatigue were caused or at least exacerbated by unrecognized long-standing depression and anxiety.

People whose pain, self-doubts, fatigue, and despair are caused by cancer—or any clearly physical illness—do not feel such guilt. They are not blamed or expected to "pull themselves together." However, if they have co-existing depression, it is likely to be overlooked. Patients with heart disease, cancer, and neurologic disorders quite often have mood disturbances (89). For example, the prevalence of major depression is six times greater in diabetics compared to the general population (86). Such patients are often thought to be simply "low" (and why not, since they are so sick?) when actually they are clinically depressed.

Many studies suggest that pre-existing clinical depression is a risk factor for heart attack and stroke. Obviously, failure to recognize true depression can have disastrous results. But psychic pain is hard to detect, and we fail to look for it when we should. Both physicians and patients tend to consider all possible "physical" causes of illness before looking at mood. One study found that 65 percent of physicians missed the presence of depression in patients with medical problems (90).

Such oversight leaves patients to suffer psychic pain and can even affect the outcome of their medical disease. The prevalence of depression is 25 percent in cancer patients and 50 percent in stroke patients (91). After a heart attack, half of patients suffer clinical depression. Of these, 75 percent remain depressed as long as a year (89). During the first six months after a heart attack, depression is an independent risk factor for death since it may cause another heart attack.

More than one million Americans are being treated for depression, but the condition is far more common than that. Studies suggest that only one in four Americans who have the illness is properly diagnosed and treated (90). Of people with syndromes like fibromyalgia, CFS, low back pain and irritable bowel syndrome, 25-50 percent have coexistent depression (15), which often goes undetected.

In recent years, the causes and therefore the treatment of major depression have begun to shift from "mental" to "physical." Formerly, the illness was believed to come entirely from environmental or experiential factors. Thus the Freudian analytic approach sought to detect and resolve these factors. Today, clinical depression is increasingly seen as a biologic disorder linked to genetic and chemical factors (92). Genes that code for improper levels of brain hormones (like serotonin; and noradrenaline) are considered the key to understanding and treating depression and other psychiatric illness (93). We cannot yet influence such genes but we have developed medications to adjust the level of brain hormones.

Among such medications are the so-called SSRIs, or selective serotonin reuptake inhibitors (92,93). As their name suggests, they target serotonin and prevent its reuptake (i.e., disappearance), making it more available to the central nervous system. Examples of these new SSRI antidepressants include Prozac, Zoloft and Paxil (Table 9). These medications are also useful for treating fibromyalgia, CFS, migraine, and irritable bowel syndrome (see Chapter 14).

In depression, such drugs are often discontinued after short-term use. They appear to be most effective when combined with psychotherapy. In my case, an antidepressant was prescribed to alleviate my depression and anxiety, along with medication to help me sleep. After about six months, I began to decrease the dosage of both and eventually discontinued them altogether. Instead of Freudian-based analysis, my psychiatrist practiced the currently more popular cognitive-behavioral therapy. Rather than searching for causes of problems in my childhood and dreams, this short-term technique focused on practical solutions. For example, the psychiatrist and I worked on specific ways to "reprogram" my reaction to stress and my preoccupation with illness.

Strange to say, despite all the positive studies and my own personal benefit, I still felt ambivalent about using antidepressant medication. My patients voice the same mixed feelings. They are often hard to convince that taking medications for depression and anxiety is as justified as taking insulin for diabetes, or thyroid hormone for the treatment of hypothyroidism. Statistics reveal that 50 percent of patients with depression do not take their prescribed drug treatment. In part, this non-compliance is due to unpleasant drug effects, but mainly it reflects guilt about taking antidepressants.

The recent media frenzy regarding Prozac has been equal parts good news and bad news. The good news, for both patients and their physicians, is that these medications are effective and have few adverse side effects. The bad news—wildly exaggerated by the media—is that Prozac has, on extremely rare occasions, led to violent behavior. The lasting negative fall-out is that many people are afraid to take this very beneficial drug.

A more rational concern is that medications like Prozac will be taken by people who are not truly ill, just to enhance their personality or productivity. Such "cosmetic psychopharmacology" might create a new age of "stressless souls," as discussed by Peter Kramer in *Listening to Prozac* (92). Kramer thoughtfully wonders whether people not suffering from pathological depression would or should take antidepressants to feel "better than well."

My own opinion is that the newer antidepressants are not likely to be gobbled by many people who do not need them. The bigger problem is that many Americans who do need these drugs are not getting them. Less than one-half of Americans with major depression are being treated. We should worry less about very rare dangers of using antidepressants than about the much larger dangers of not using them.

At the same time, we must beware of the pitfalls inherant with relying only on drugs or on physicians. In his book <u>Speaking of Sadness</u>, David Karp discusses his own use of medications to treat depression (94). A professor of sociology at Boston College, he offers a perspective on illness and society that differs in interesting ways from mine. Karp writes that taking antidepressants conjured up in him "a mixture of hostility and dependence." He distrusts the purely biochemical explanation of depression as much too simple. It ignores the effect of our surroundings on mind and body that, as a sociologist, he appreciates very well.

Most of all, Karp is concerned about the medical tendency to separate illness from the person who is ill. This is never a good thing but may be especially serious with regard to depression. For all of us, the impact of any disease or illness is determined by our interaction with everything and everyone in our life. The biologic basis for depression must be recognized so medications can play their role in treatment. But its non-biologic aspects must be also remembered and given the attention they need.

If personal problems or crises pile up, driving us from normal discouragement to debilitating depression, medication is not the whole answer. It may roll back the depression, but cannot tend to the conditions that brought it on. Those problems and crises need human care and caring from physicians, friends and family.

SECTION III:
RESOLVING OPPOSING VIEWS OF THESE ILLNESSES

Chapter 10:
Finding a cause—the patient's response

Every spring, as a child, I would be miserable with sniffling and coughing. Our family doctor would give me a shot of penicillin that never seemed to help. In medical school I was diagnosed with multiple allergies and received injections to "desensitize" me. These were very effective, but whenever I got a viral or bacterial infection, my allergy symptoms flared up for weeks. In recent years, these allergies led to bacterial sinus infections and extreme fatigue.

Surgery helped, but finally I was diagnosed with asthma. Inhalers were prescribed, but I kept wheezing until placed on prednisone. This helped a lot, but I worried about the side effects of such corticosteroids, which I knew all too well from my patients. I wondered why in the world I was plagued with all these ailments. Maybe there was something really wrong with my immune system. I had AIDS testing, since I had once been stuck with a needle while drawing blood from a patient. Results were negative. Then I began to wonder about the air supply in our new office. Could our medical building have the "the sick building syndrome"?

Testing by an environmental expert found no evidence of toxins, but this did not alleviate my concern. Like anyone else with a health mystery, I wanted a solution. Even when our illness has a cure, we want to know the *cause*. We want to get better but also want to *stay better*, by avoiding whatever made us sick in the first place. Clearly infections and allergens can cause illness. However, one person may become sick when exposed, while the next person remains healthy. I was convinced that I was excessively susceptible to infections.

Germs are the "agents of disease" but individuals vary widely in their inherent susceptibility (95). Our personal vulnerability is determined by many factors that determine the state of our physical and mental health. As has been said many times in this book, our mind and body—not one or the other—determine how we react to infection or to any other stressor.

Typically, infections come and go with no lingering effect. When we get the flu, its effects on the nervous system produce fatigue, muscle aches, headaches, disturbed sleep, and bowel irritability. We feel depressed, irritable, and have trouble concentrating, but are usually back to our old selves in a few days. However, such symptoms persist indefinitely in chronic disorders like fibromyalgia and CFS. Often, the most disturbing symptom is the fatigue, which people describe as "waves of exhaustion." You feel leaden and lethargic. You want to sleep all the time, and you doze off a lot—but nighttime sleep is never refreshing. You ache all over.

What is going on here? The fact is that while most infections come and go, we sometimes see two kinds of lasting effect. Everyone knows, for example, that polio can damage the nervous system to cause permanent paralysis. Less well known is that almost any kind of infection may cause lasting damage by activating immune or inflammatory factors. Long after the infection has run its course, such activation can cause ongoing or recurrent illness.

A good example is Lyme disease, so-called because its first reported cases occurred near Lyme, Connecticut. Its bacterial agent, a new discovery, is associated with direct tissue invasion and straightforward symptoms. But it is also associated with chronic illness and symptoms that lack a clear cause or cure.

The Lyme microbe enters the skin during a tick bite (which can generally be avoided by staying out of underbrush or wearing protective clothing). It may work its way into joint tissue, causing arthritic pain and swelling. Or it can enter the nervous system and cause paralysis of the seventh cranial nerve (Bell's palsy) or other neurologic symptoms. In either case, symptoms are directly traceable to tissue invasion. Such symptoms can usually be alleviated by antibiotic treatment.

However, as in the next case, a Lyme infection that has supposedly been eradicated can be followed by fatigue, pain, and problems with concentration.

Betsy: Lyme disease and chronic neurologic problems

Betsy consulted me because of three years of chronic muscle and joint pain and persistent fatigue. In the spring of 1993, when vacationing in northern New England, she developed a large, circular rash on her right thigh. Although she did not remember a tick bite, she had been walking through a marsh where Lyme disease had been reported. During the next few days, Betsy had a low-grade fever, felt very tired and achy, and had a sore right knee. She saw a general physician who told her that the rash was characteristic of that seen in the earliest stages of Lyme disease. A blood test confirmed a recent Lyme infection. He prescribed a two-week course of antibiotics.

During the next few weeks, Betsy gradually felt better. Her fever and skin rash disappeared and never returned. However, over the next 6 months, Betsy experienced constant muscle and joint pains, but no swelling. She had persistent fatigue, but could not sleep well during the night. Along with headaches that worsened, she began having dizziness and mental confusion.

A specialist was consulted and told Betsy that he suspected central nervous system Lyme disease. To determine whether there were bacteria in the brain and spinal fluid, Betsy underwent 2 spinal taps, an EEG, a brain and spinal cord MRI, and multiple blood tests. All results were normal but, because of the possibility that Betsy had persistent Lyme infection of the nervous system, she was placed on a month-long course of intravenous antibiotics. During that month, she felt slightly more energetic but over the next year the muscle pains, fatigue, headaches and cognitive disturbances persisted. Last year, she had another 4-week trial of a different and "stronger" antibiotic. She noted no improvement.

When I evaluated Betsy, she continued to have severe fatigue and muscle pain. Her physical examination was unremarkable except for extreme tenderness over the fibromyalgia "tender points." Her neurologic examination was normal. The blood tests demonstrated that she had been infected with the Lyme bacteria in the past, but further tests demonstrated no evidence for persistent, active infection. I told Betsy that she had a fibromyalgia/chronic fatigue syndrome that might have been triggered by the Lyme infection. But I doubted that her symptoms were caused by a current Lyme infection. I began her on a low dose of amitriptyline at bedtime which helped her to sleep better and improved her muscle pain. During the next 6 months, she gradually felt less exhaustion, and the headaches and dizziness disappeared. She was relieved to be told that her brain was not harboring an infection that no one had eradicated.

Lyme disease can easily be confused with fibromyalgia and CFS because they share similar symptoms. However, the classic skin rash and joint swelling of Lyme disease are not found in fibromyalgia and CFS. Blood tests for Lyme disease may be negative despite an active infection (a "false negative" result), but this is rare.

Most people who have been treated with antibiotics for suspected Lyme disease *without improvement* probably never had Lyme disease at all. They more likely had fibromyalgia and chronic fatigue, which are much more common than Lyme disease. Even where Lyme disease is endemic, such as New England, fewer than .01 percent of the population (one in 10,000) ever develop the disease. Five to ten percent of the population have fibromyalgia and chronic fatigue.

However, it is crucial to point out that many people in such areas have been *exposed* to the Lyme agent, which caused unnoticed infection. Many agents can cause infection without disease. Furthermore, some microbes set up permanent housekeeping in the human body and even work for us. But good or bad, transient or permanent, such colonizers cause our immune system to generate antibodies. Therefore, if people previously exposed to Lyme disease eventually suffer some illness that suggests Lyme disease, they will be tested and found "positive." This "false positive" antibody test result may lead to treatment for Lyme disease that is useless and ignores their real problem. To avoid this mistake, physicians should perform Lyme antibody tests only in patients with signs and symptoms that are clinically suggestive of Lyme disease.

Another reason for confusion of Lyme disease with syndromes like fibromyalgia and CFS is that such syndromes can arise during—or shortly after—the course of a Lyme infection. In such cases, people develop Lyme infection that is appropriately treated and "cured" with antibiotics. Then, like Betsy, they continue to have symptoms of chronic pain, fatigue, sleep and mood disturbances (44). In the vast majority of these cases, extensive studies have failed to find any evidence of continuing

Lyme infection. Repeated courses of antibiotics do no good.

In such cases, Lyme infection appears to have triggered chronic illness with neurologic and musculoskeletal symptoms. These are sometimes called "post-Lyme disease," but the symptoms are identical to those of fibromyalgia and CFS.

So an infection like Lyme disease can cause illness in the classic medical model, but also may trigger a chronic syndrome by uncertain pathways. Similarly, allergens can play a dual role. However, confusion and controversy have developed because people confuse true allergens with other types of irritants in our food or environment. In this area, as throughout this book, I have sadly learned from personal experience.

In addition to my allergies to pollens, grass and trees, I have sensitivities to certain foods. For example, I get a headache and diarrhea from eating food that contains monosodium glutamate (MSG). Patty has a similar reaction to milk or other products containing lactose. These very common reactions are termed individual hypersensitivities. They are very annoying and can mimic allergies in their symptoms. They can contribute to the gastroabdominal distress of such problems as irritable bowel syndrome. However, they are not immune-mediated allergies, such as hay fever. They do not arise from the immune system or permanently affect that system. They do not, in themselves, cause chronic illness.

Many non-traditional health care practitioners and their books claim that certain foods or environmental substances cause many chronic illnesses and symptoms. For example, sugar and certain food additives have been blamed for hyperactivity in children. After much controversy, this idea has been largely discredited by scientific testing. Unfortunately, people who hear and believe such unfounded theories seem rarely to hear the scientific evidence against them. In part this is because the media gives more attention to "newsworthy" theories than to workaday science. Also, not knowing how it works, many people seem to distrust science. Yet with all its flaws (and the flaws of scientists, who are only human), science is our best way to separate truth from half-truth or sheer fiction.

Non-traditional practitioners also attribute chronic illness to chemicals in our environment. We have all experienced distress when exposed to noxious irritants such as smoke, car exhaust fumes, ammonia, pesticides, paint, and glue. People vary in such sensitivity, but even the most extreme distress does not represent a classic allergy. It has nothing to do with immune hypersensitivity. Yet many patients are quite certain that their chronic illness was caused by some environmental exposure.

Diane: Allergies and chemical sensitivity

Diane is a 29-year-old female who was well until two years ago. At that time she was working as an administrative assistant in a large law firm. She had a history of allergies to grass and trees and suffered from asthma as a child. Two years ago she began getting recurrent colds, sore throats, and runny nose. A number of other workers on her floor had similar symptoms and eventually there was concern that the ventilation system in the building was causing these reactions. An environmental analysis found unacceptable levels of certain chemicals in the building and the ventilation system was overhauled. However, Diane's allergic symptoms worsened and she began getting severe headaches, shortness of breath, and unusual hive-like rashes within two hours of coming to work. She also had two bouts of bacterial sinus infection (sounds familiar to me!) which were successfully treated with long courses of antibiotics. Except for these two infections, her physicians could find no cause of her symptoms despite a very complete evaluation.

Over the next six months, she developed progressively worse nasal congestion, wheezing, and cough, plus diarrhea and nausea. She became very fatigued, had difficulty falling asleep and trouble concentrating. Her appetite disappeared, and many foods that she used to enjoy caused either diarrhea or constipation. She lost 15 pounds over 6 months. She then took a leave of absence from work. After seeing two pulmonary and Ear, Nose and Throat specialists who also found "no physical problems," her primary physician suggested that she see a psychiatrist. The patient was very upset with the implication that her symptoms were "not real." She sought help from a holistic physician who directed an "allergy-immunology clinic." There she was told that her blood tests and skin tests demonstrated allergies to a large number of pollens, foods, and chemicals. She also was told that her blood tests showed antibodies to the Epstein-Barr virus, other viruses, and Candida (yeast). Based on these tests she was diagnosed to have Multiple Chemical Sensitivity Syndrome and Chronic Fatigue Immune Dysfunction Syndrome.

Diane was then started on a strict "elimination diet" and also given injections of tiny amounts of allergens to "desensitize" her system. She was also treated with a number of herbal and natural substances. The non-traditional physician told Diane that this therapy would bolster her failing immune system. However, her symptoms did not get better and she became more limited in her lifestyle. Eventually, she could not go out of her house because she feared that exposure to fumes such as smoke or perfume would aggravate her symptoms.

After evaluating Diane, I agreed that she had a history of classic pollen-induced allergies. In fact, 10-15 percent of the population is allergic to ragweed and other plant pollens. Other common allergens include animal dander, dust, dust mites, and wood products. Reactions caused by such allergens trigger the body to produce excess immunoglobulin E (IgE), which stimulates mast cells and other cells. These cells in turn secrete substances like histamine that produce the typical symptoms affecting the nose, throat, eyes, lungs, and skin. Certain skin-prick tests and blood tests confirm such immune-related reactions and distinguish them from hypersensitivities not related to the immune system.

I also agreed that antibodies to pathogens like Epstein-Barr virus proved previous infection. However, I stressed that such positive tests do not prove ongoing infection, in the absense of any symptoms of infection. Nor do they prove infection-related effects on the immune system.

Many of Diane's symptoms, such as the fatigue, sleep and memory problems, suggested fibromyalgia and chronic fatigue syndrome. There is much similarity between those syndromes and what has been termed the "multiple chemical sensitivity syndrome" (96). I could not argue that some substance in her workplace might have been a factor in her illness. However, I was concerned that Diane perceived as allergens some substances that were not allergens. More important, I felt her perception—and her efforts to avoid these substances—had caused great stress on her. It was complicating her recovery and the conduct of her life. She had become fearful of eating, drinking, or going out anywhere.

Patients with symptoms like Diane's are often told by alternative therapists that they have a chronic infection or a serious immunologic problem caused by chemicals. Advised to rest and avoid the "chemicals," they may become very hesitant about participating in normal activities. Diane had always enjoyed aerobics, tennis, and skiing, but had gradually stopped all forms of exercise and became increasingly deconditioned. She felt helpless because of the conviction that her illness was due to infection or to immune dysfunction over which she had no control. The elimination diet greatly restricted her food intake and made her worry about the hundreds of potential "allergens" in her diet and environment. This contributed to her alarming weight loss.

Diane was diagnosed to have multiple chemical sensitivity syndrome by a physician called a clinical ecologist. Such specialists focus on environmental illnesses including the candidiasis hypersensitivity syndrome (popularly known as "The Yeast Connection"), total allergy syndrome, and chemically induced immune dysregulation. They contend that many illnesses—from cancer to chronic fatigue syndrome—are caused by chemicals in the air that we breathe or the food that we eat. They postulate that "environmental illnesses" derive from the failure of humans to adapt to today's profusion of synthetic chemicals. In some individuals, they say, the immune system is overwhelmed by a kind of chemical overload. Patients suspected of such overload are tested to determine specific sensitivities or "allergens." These substances are then gradually eliminated from the person's diet or surroundings.

Some truth may hide among all these theories, but so far they are only theories. The tests used by clinical ecologists—and other such health advocates—have not been accepted by most traditional physicians. They do not give consistent results because they have not been standardized. While intense exposure to irritants can be risky, no scientific evidence has shown that brief and incidental exposure can lead to chronic poor health.

Told they are "allergic" to hundreds of substances, patients like Diane face an impossible living situation. A few years ago, on an episode from the television program "Northern Exposure," an intelligent and wealthy young man was preoccupied by his multiple chemical sensitivities. He built himself an environmentally "safe" home in Alaska. It was shielded from electromagnetic waves. His air and water supplies were meticulously filtered. The food was "de-contaminated," and he strictly adhered to a diet that avoided all synthetic additives. His anxiety about joining the community and establishing a relationship with Maggie, the female lead, reminded me of Diane.

I explained to her that none of my thousands of patients with fibromyalgia, CFS, or irritable bowel syndrome had evidence of significant immune deficiency. Evidence to the contrary was provided by testing and by the fact that no one developed immune-related malignancies or infections such as AIDS.

I agreed that many of her symptoms could have been triggered or aggravated by infections or her response to the environment. However, I could not agree that her chronic fatigue, rashes, and gastrointestinal symptoms could all be eliminated by an ecology treatment program. This pushed speculation and scientific uncertainty into a realm of unfounded half-truths. Even if environmental factors were to damage the immune system, removing such factors would not be likely to undo the damage. Once Diane understood this, she was much better able to get on with her life.

We should certainly consider the possibility that environmental irritants are detrimental to our health. What could be clearer than smoking causing cancer? I do not doubt that people have reactions to various irritants. Indeed, I'm convinced that my frequent airplane trips have aggravated my sinus infections. Scientific evidence shows that people with upper airway hypersensitivity are prone to such infections, which will often trigger more allergic symptoms or asthma. Most specialists agree that our rising rates of asthma and allergies reflect the rising level of contaminants in our air, water, and food supply. We should continue to research the possibility that our environment impacts many chronic illnesses and work politically for a cleaner living environment.

Allergies are common in patients with fibromyalgia and CFS. Migraine headaches have also been linked to allergies. I am interested in evidence that certain mind-body treatments can be useful in treating certain allergies; that acupuncture and relaxation techniques can help alleviate allergic upper respiratory symptoms. My own team of professionals includes a physician who sometimes uses the principles of acupuncture.

What I cannot accept, without more evidence, is that dietary or environmental substances *cause* syndromes like fibromyalgia. I cannot accept many "treatments" that are based on little or no scientific evaluation. I do not believe that patients suffering chronic illness benefit from untested approaches that make them more fearful and preoccupied with their health problems. If they sometimes *appear* to benefit in the short term, I strongly suspect coincidence or the placebo effect.

Most of all, I object to patient "advocates" or health care professionals who "have all the answers." I object to the millions of dollars generated by the growing "health press" and the "alternative medicine" that offer cures for syndromes like fibromyalgia, CFS, migraine, low back pain, and depression—not to mention diseases like cancer, diabetes, and arthritis.

An alternative medicine journal, published this year, urged people to "treat your fibroids without surgery" or try "homeopathic relief for toothache." It claimed that "asthmatics tend to have a 50 percent lower blood concentration of vitamin C than healthy people." It told readers to "skip the Valium, hold the Prozac, but instead bolster your amino acid reserves." These reserves can be determined by "electro-dermal screening" or "hair analysis." Then you can order products with good solid American marketing names like "Vital Force," exotic names like ashwagandha, and Latin-sounding names like boswellia, lactospore, and curcuminoids. You can order the cheerfully named "Despondency," a preparation described as "a safe, natural remedy for emotional burnout and mental exhaustion."

These outrageous claims are the worst kind of hucksterism. They prey on people's fears and insecurities, waste their money, and sometimes endanger their health. To mislead the public that "PhytoSOY" will "stop aging and degeneration" is bad enough. Far worse are alternative cancer treatments such as "ukrain," "iscador", "carnivora" and "glandular extracts." Such products take advantage of desperation. They promote false hope and are sometimes actually harmful in their contents. They are most harmful in keeping a patient from trying a traditional cancer treatment that might be life-saving.

We all want causes and cures for our problems—including my sinus infections!—but we must be armed with skepticism, common sense, and good judgment as we continue to be bombarded by unfounded claims.

Chapter 11:
Finding a disease: The medical profession's response

Physicians are trained in the scientific method, which requires objective evidence to diagnose a disease. To qualify, the disease must have verifiable pathologic and physiologic cause, signs, and course of development, as in pneumonia or heart disease. Unfortunately, many chronic illnesses do not meet these requirements, and are thus viewed with skepticism by the medical profession.

Many health care practitioners prefer to think of fibromyalgia, migraine, chronic fatigue syndrome, irritable bowel syndrome, depression, and low back pain as transient episodes within a *normal* state of health. They argue that the most healthy person has ups and downs, suffering occasional aches and pains, fatigue, insomnia, blue days, or headaches. Therefore, syndromes with such symptoms do not necessarily reflect poor health; they more likely reflect a *poor individual response* to normal health and the normal hardships of life.

A Boston <u>Globe</u> health column (June 3, 1996) discussed fibromyalgia, CFS, multiple chemical sensitivity syndrome and attention deficit disorder as "fad illnesses." It quoted medical experts who believed some of these conditions to be "genuine" but "greatly over-diagnosed."

The experts complained that the symptoms of these illnesses are non-specific and overlapping; that patients and practitioners too often resort to the latest "fad illness" label; that sometimes such labels obscure "real problems" that go untreated.

I disagree: these illnesses are indeed real problems. They are more likely to be underdiagnosed than overdiagnosed. However, one neurologist asserts a more negative opinion: that fibromyalgia is nothing more than hypervigilance and somatoform pain. This is current medical jargon for what used to be called hypochondriasis and hysteria (97). In short, it is all in the head. This physician even suggests that fibromyalgia represents collusion of medical and legal interests for financial gain.

A prominent rheumatologist equates fibromyalgia with being "out of sorts"(98). He says that we all have bad days characterized by stiffness and achiness, easy fatigue, loss of well-being, and preoccupation with our bowels. He claims that the diagnosis of fibromyalgia does harm because assigning a label to the normal hardships of life "teaches people to be sick." Similarly, an Australian physician says that terms like "fibromyalgia" promote abnormal illness behavior, which is then reinforced by societal provision of advantages for the sick (99). He states that pain is not "organic" unless accompanied by pathophysiologic abnormalities. In other words, pain without objective evidence is psychological.

I strongly disagree that a diagnosis of fibromyalgia encourages illness or illness behavior. Yet this is a common belief with regard to many syndromes, including CFS. Abbey and Garfinkel (100) have traced the history of neurasthenia and CFS in Western society. They consider them the same phenomenon and ascribe both to times preoccupied with material success. Such times have seen major role changes for women, who therefore suffer unusual stress. For the nineteenth century physician, this resulted in a "depletion of our limited supply of nervous energy" (a literal translation of "neurasthenia"). Abbey and Garfinkel believe that a diagnosis of CFS legitimizes dubious symptoms and promotes illness behavior, sickness behavior and abandonment of the workplace. They predict that "chronic fatigue syndrome" is a fad label that will fade away, as did neurasthenia.

The same debate surrounds the diagnostic labels of migraine and depression. However, these two disorders, once blamed entirely on stress, are now widely accepted to have a biological basis. With migraine, this involves complicated genetic, vascular, and hormonal interactions. As these interactions are better understood, more specific medications to treat migraine are becoming available. Likewise, depression is now well characterized as a discrete syndrome with a genetic and neurohormonal basis that responds to specific treatment. The progress on these two disorders suggests that further research may well reveal important biologic components to fibromyalgia and CFS.

However, some skeptics still ignore the biologic basis of depression. To them, it is an "illness" only because some of their colleagues have labeled normal states of unhappiness as a medical disorder. David Karp deplores the "medicalization of society" that makes normalcy a synonym for health and abnormalcy a synonym for pathology (94). He points to cultural and generational differences in the perception and labeling of illness. In modern China, for example, "mental illness" is so stigmatizing that the diagnosis is virtually non-existent. Interestingly, the Chinese resort to the old-fashioned diagnosis of neurasthenia when people suffer symptoms of depression, anxiety, fatigue, headaches, and insomnia.

Thus the medical profession is divided in regard to the very existence of these syndromes. Physicians who doubt they are discrete entities argue that the symptoms have no organic basis, they cannot be verified by tests, nor can they be treated successfully. Such physicians tend to think that giving a name like "fibromyalgia" to these common symptoms encourages people to think they are ill when, in fact, they are only having a normal period of "unwellness."

A "gender bias" no doubt plays a part in this debate. Fibromyalgia, chronic fatigue syndrome, migraine, irritable bowel syndrome, and depression are all more common in women than in men. This confirms the belief held by some physicians that women, more than men, tend to react psychosomatically when life is hard. It could more cogently be argued that such illness is related to hormonal factors in women. It may even be related to the stress of living in a male-dominated society where female problems are brushed aside. Yet I too often hear from my colleagues that women with these syndromes simply need a "stiff upper lip."

The gender bias is perhaps most clearly revealed in debates about the diagnosis and treatment of premenstrual syndrome (PMS). PMS shares many symptoms with fibromyalgia and CFS, though it is most noted for irritability and other mood disturbances. A recent placebo-controlled medication trial found that PMS symptoms were alleviated by Prozac (101). For physicians who see Prozac as simply a tranquilizer, this trial was "evidence" that PMS is a stress response typical of women, especially certain "personality types." However, a more scientific interpretation is that Prozac alleviates PMS because it acts on observable biologic phenomena. The response of PMS to a specific serotonin reuptake inhibitor, such as Prozac, shows that serotonin is a factor in PMS mood and appetite disturbances. PMS thus appears to be less a function of female "weakness" than to changes in female chemistry related to the menstrual cycle.

Are fibromyalgia and similar syndromes best seen as "illness" or as normal episodes of poor health? Wellness

and illness cannot be clearly separated because they oc-
cupy a continuum. I define these syndromes as "illness"
because, although their symptoms occur in healthy people, they occur here at a persistent and debilitating level.
People who suffer these symptoms on a chronic basis
represent a well-defined group. They may not have a
medical "disease," but they are plagued by significant ill-
health, or *illness.* Their syndromes may be diagnosed on
the basis of clear and established criteria.

To label a set of symptoms as a syndrome benefits most
people by offering a diagnosis, support and alleviating
uncertainty. Most of us with chronic pain, headaches, fatigue, or depression do not want to be ill. We have become
"ill" or "patients" long before we are diagnosed with any
syndrome. The diagnostic label is a great relief. It gives us
hope and lifts fears of much worse disorders. A diagnosis
of fibromyalgia is a relief to the patient who fears lupus,
for example, or the migraine patient who fears a brain
tumor. The earlier the diagnosis, the better, because it
saves costly testing and needless worry. One study
showed that patients with a diagnosis of fibromyalgia
were ten times less likely to be hospitalized than similar
patients with no diagnosis (102).

An interesting study compares the views of doctors
and patients as to the value of a CFS diagnosis (103).
Seventy percent of general practitioners were reluctant to
make a diagnosis of CFS. They felt "constrained by the
scientific uncertainty regarding the cause of CFS" and
concerned that the diagnosis might become a self-fulfill-
ing prophecy. In contrast, patients thought that the diagnosis of CFS was "enabling" because it provided a coh-
erent explanation for their illness.

In my experience, most patients with these chronic
illnesses improve once they are given a diagnosis and
treatment plan. Most go on to lead a much more normal
life, even if their chronic symptoms remain. Treatment of

fibromyalgia, irritable bowel syndrome, migraine, and depression is generally quite helpful despite rarely being a "cure." Even this level of treatment would not be available if these syndromes had not been defined.

Whether healthy people sometimes suffer these symptoms is hardly germane to the 5-20 percent of people whose suffering has reached the point of chronic illness. Even when—or perhaps especially when—a "disease" cannot be identified, it cannot hurt patients to assign a label. In fact, it helps them—by telling them they are not crazy: their illness is real and shared by many other people. Their symptoms may be "normal," but their suffering is well beyond the "norm." Their symptoms have reached a level of poor health that needs medical care.

Hypertension offers an apt analogy. We all vary in our blood pressure, and a healthy person may occasionally have a dramatic rise in blood pressure as a response to stress. Whether or not we have hypertension that requires medical treatment depends on how much and how often our blood pressure is beyond the established "norm" for the population. If it is seriously beyond, the condition is seen as a disease that requires vigorous treatment. But what about mild or borderline hypertension? Is it a disease, an illness, or something less? Should it be labeled and treated? Many patients with mild hypertension could live with their condition, untreated, especially if they lost weight and made other lifestyle changes. A few who are "labeled" with hypertension will exaggerate their problem in unfortunate ways. However, most of those patients are better off knowing they have an illness that can—and should be—controlled. Most physicians will put such patients on medication and check them regularly. These patients will have a better life and live longer because they were diagnosed and treated.

Chapter 12:
Finding a balance: Accepting uncertainty and mind-body interactions

The symptoms that we have been exploring are sometimes signs of a serious disease. Before settling on a
diagnosis of fibromyalgia or CFS, the physician must exclude diseases like cancer, lupus, and multiple sclerosis.
Usually this is easily done, but patients may insist that
disease is lurking somewhere. They are often dissatisfied
with the notion that nothing can be found. I myself was
hard to convince. I needed time and help to accept the
uncertainties of my illness and health. Some patients, like
the following, are even harder to convince.

Emma: Diagnostic uncertainty and chronic illness

*Emma, a 49-year-old female, reported a history of not feeling
well since age 35. Her symptoms included fatigue, intermittent
joint and muscle aches, skin rashes, sensitivity to many foods
and perfumes, allergies, diarrhea and constipation. At age 36,
she had a single blood test that was positive for lupus (systemic
lupus erythematosus). She was told that she might eventually
develop lupus, and became very concerned about this possibility.
Over the next 5 years she had seen 5 different rheumatologists*

and 4 immunologists. No exact diagnosis of lupus or any other disease had been made.

In more recent years, Emma complained of increasing problems with her concentration, heart palpitations, numbness and tingling over her arms and legs, and problems with her balance. She had been evaluated by four different neurologists. Two told her that there was nothing physically wrong and that her symptoms were "all in your head." Two told her that she may have early multiple sclerosis. She had undergone 5 MRI's of the brain and spine during the past 5 years. Emma denied feeling depressed but admitted to extreme anxiety regarding her health and the absence of a specific diagnosis.

Over the next 3 years Emma made many visits to numerous specialists and was admitted to the hospital four times because of chest pain and palpitations. Her cardiac evaluation was normal each time. When her primary physician recommended that she see a psychiatrist, she became very upset and angry. She thought that he was refusing to believe that her symptoms were real and telling her that, after all this time, she was just a hypochondriac. She nevertheless saw the psychiatrist. He told her that she did not demonstrate evidence for a psychiatric illness, but was very anxious and would probably benefit from treatment for the anxiety. Emma refused to start medications for anxiety or to accept counseling.

Patients with chronic illness often consult with many physicians and specialists in search of answers. Since the world's wisest specialist cannot know everything, this makes sense up to a point. If prolonged, however, this search becomes the kind of "doctor shopping" that is an end in itself. It keeps patients from accepting uncertainty and shifting their focus to feeling better.

I finally convinced Emma that her symptoms were real but not a sign of severe disease. She was then able to deal more effectively with her anxiety, but her uncertainties continue to plague her. They make her very reluctant to participate in many normal activities for fear they might aggravate her symptoms. I can certainly sympathize. It was a struggle for me to realize that I could achieve a positive impact on my illnesses even if their "cause" was never found.

Most people don't fret over a rare and fleeting episode of illness. But if ill repeatedly or over a long period, they want to know why. It seems logical to blame an injury or infection. Most patients with chronic back or neck pain blame an injury, often minor and many years past. According to scientific evidence, chronic muscular pain cannot in most cases be traced to such injury. Yet societal and financial pressures cause patients to pursue the myth. Practitioners add fuel by talking of "misalignments" that must be "fixed" by manipulation or surgery. Alternatively, they prescribe rest or a splint for the involved joint or muscle, which promotes inactivity—the worst course in most cases (Figure 1).

For centuries, the problems now called fibromyalgia were blamed on physical abnormalities in the muscle. We now know that the structure and function of the muscle is normal in fibromyalgia. This is important for patients to accept because, if concerned about a muscle injury, they resist the moderate exercise that will do them the most good. Similarly, patients with CFS need to know that its extreme fatigue has no verifiable cause, though some physicians still blame a virus or other infection (48). The fatigue responds better to more activity than to more rest.

Of course, most people with chronic pain and fatigue don't want to hear that we do not know the cause of their illness. They may feel that the medical establishment is brushing aside their claims and concerns. They can be very sensitive when physicians mention the role of stress and mood. Even when the reference is sympathetic and refers to the mind-body connection, they hear "it's all in your head." Such physicians are rejected as "not listening to me."

The challenge facing clinicians and scientists is to keep listening. Although we have not confirmed a direct link of fibromyalgia and CFS to an infection, injury, or the environment, we must keep searching. After all, illnesses long felt to have a largely psychologic basis have turned out to have a classic biomedical cause. The most recent example is peptic ulcer disease. For centuries, it was thought to be caused by excess stomach acid production in response to stress. We prescribed antacids and told patients to reduce their stress levels. Suddenly, the organism *Helicobacter pylori* was revealed as the culprit in many cases. Now we treat most ulcers with antibiotics, a course that ten years ago would have been unthinkable.

We must hope that the near future will bring more exact understanding of the cause or causes of fibromyalgia, CFS, migraine, and depression. Until then, physicians must stretch to become more open-minded about these problems. Patients must stretch to accept that, at least for now, their symptoms have no cause or cure. If both sides stretch, they can find a balanced approach to management of chronic illness. Patients can better cope and get on with their lives.

Unfortunately the balance will always be fragile and threatened at times by the media. When science announces a new finding, the media too often behaves as if it is the "last word." It tends to applaud each yet-to-be-proven theory, then attack when problems arise. This unrealistic approach to the workings of science has sadly led to distrust of the medical profession. People run to their doctor about the latest sensational "cure" and are frustrated to find it unavailable. The doctor too often adds to their frustration by not taking time to explain the situation. Too often physicians act as if patients have no right to question the medical establishment. Rights aside, patients *will question* and doctors must try to answer, if only to counter media disinformation. The old "no comment" response to patients or media will only create more distrust.

The continuing furor over silicone breast-implants shows what can happen when media and public decide on a "cause" for illness, without benefit of science. Many women believe the implants have caused fibromyalgia and other types of chronic illness.

Tammy: Silicone breast implant and chronic illness

Tammy is a 48-year-old female who began experiencing bouts of fatigue 7 years ago. Since that time she "always had poor energy" and reported difficulty recovering from viral or bacterial infections. Four years ago she began having daily headaches. Her physician found no abnormalities on physical examination or laboratory testing. She had resigned herself to the fact that she was "just a low energy person." Then she read a newspaper report suggesting a link between chronic ill health and silicone breast implants. Tammy had silicone breast implants inserted when she was age 25. They had not bothered her, as far as she knew. However, her fatigue and other symptoms were similar to symptoms described in the media as related to implants.

During the next 2 years she saw numerous physicians to find out if she had implant-related health problems. Although there were no abnormalities in her immunologic blood tests, one of four "experts" told her she had signs of silicone-induced immune disease, which he termed "siliconosis." He recommended that the implants be removed. She became very nervous about this decision, losing sleep over it during the next 6 months. Eventually, the implants were removed.

When I examined Tammy 6 months later, she was still complaining of bouts of severe fatigue. She was involved in class-action litigation against the manufacturer of her silicone breast implants. Her medical evaluation demonstrated no evidence of an immunologic disorder or any connective tissue disease. However, Tammy firmly believed that her illness was caused by the implants and was very angry at the medical profession for "lying to me."

More than one million women in the United States had silicone breast implants inserted between 1964 and 1992 (104). The implants were considered to be safe, although at least 20 percent leaked into the surrounding breast tissue, causing poor cosmetic results. Beginning in the 1980s, a series of medical reports suggested that the implants might cause immune diseases such as lupus or scleroderma.

When scientists report early results in a new investigation, other scientists view the findings as preliminary. They know they are not the last word. However, the media and public often lack this perspective. So before the reports on the implants could be substantiated by further studies, women began to bring suit and plaintiffs began to receive large sums of money for compensation.

On April 16, 1992, the U.S. Food and Drug Administration hastily banned the use of silicone gel-filled breast implants. The FDA hedged by stating that there was no data linking implants to any systemic disease, but that manufacturers had not tested enough to prove safety. The media then uncovered evidence that certain manufacturers of implants had falsified potentially damaging results in early testing. This fed suspicion that the FDA knew implants were unsafe but was "covering" to protect its reputation or the interests of implant manufacturers. Outrage over implant safety now exploded, as did lawsuits filed against the implant manufacturers. Awards of $5-7 millions were given to some women who had very nonspecific complaints attributed to the implants. Most of these women had neither lupus nor scleroderma.

Finally, but much too late, a number of epidemiologic studies were designed and carried out specifically to determine, once and for all, whether silicone breast implants could cause systemic connective tissue disease. They found no clear evidence to support this idea (105,106). One study found what appeared to be a very small increased risk (107). In that report, 1 percent of all women developed a connective-tissue disease, compared with 2 percent in women with breast implants. This is "double the risk," which makes a good headline! Yet the risk is still minuscule, as readers learn if a news story provides the percentages. Unfortunately, the most responsible media often use an eye-catching headline and provide the figures late in the story, if at all. Readers who skim can get a skewed impression, so when following scientific news, be sure to read the whole story!

The above studies suggest that the vast majority of women who become ill after receiving a breast implant do not have a diagnosable "disease" caused by the implant. However, the public remains suspicious. Patient advocacy groups and lawyers have attacked the "negative" studies. They have even suggested that results were manipulated to hide a link between implants and disease, given the fact that some studies were partially funded by makers of implants.

Such attacks sadly show how little the public trusts or understands science. These studies were performed by some of the finest epidemiologists in the country, including several at Harvard Medical School and the Mayo Clinic. Such investigators would not risk their credibility to profit from studies. Nor *could* they profit, since funding does not depend in any way on the results. Meanwhile, despite the absence of scientific evidence that implants cause systemic disease, billions of dollars are being awarded to women who claim that their illness is related to the implants.

It is important to note that most of these women are indeed "ill." They most commonly suffer fibromyalgia and chronic fatigue syndrome (108). Therefore, silicone breast implants, just like infections (Lyme disease or viral disease), physical trauma and emotional trauma, may trigger a chronic stress reaction leading to one of these common, chronic illnesses. However, this does not establish cause and effect, nor does it implicate implants in causing diseases like lupus or scleroderma.

Unfortunately, the silicone breast controversy has pitted medicine against the public. Women with implants have become victims of the controversy, whether there is truth in it or not. These women are frightened about their future health and uncertain whether their implants should be removed. Many have become anxious and depressed, and some have completely lost trust in their physicians. Physicians, attorneys and the media should all reexamine their role in this fiasco.

One problem that seems to plague American society is an unrealistic desire for certainty. Our media continually encourages and exploits this, as shown in the Kevorkian case mentioned earlier in this book. Two contrasting stories appeared in Boston newspapers when Dr. Kevorkian assisted the suicide of the Massachusetts woman who had fibromyalgia and CFS. The more responsible story used the headline, "Doctors say her case treatable, nonfatal." It focused on whether physician-assisted suicide is morally justified when the potential suicide victim has a non-fatal disease. Four medical experts, including myself, were quoted to verify that fibromyalgia and CFS are not fatal, and that treatment for these illnesses is generally helpful although not curative. This story used the Kevorkian incident to give the public some useful information.

The less responsible story was headlined, "Docs clash over suicide, autopsy." It focused on the medical profession's inability to properly diagnose and treat disorders like CFS. Two attorneys and one patient with CFS were quoted, but no medical experts. The story suggested that CFS and fibromyalgia are degenerative, are caused by viruses, and result in brain abnormalities revealed by MRI or SPECT scans. Not one of these assertions is supported by strong scientific evidence! This story sought not to inform but to stir up the public. Its account of the case led to many of my own patients expressing new fears and confusion.

Medicine, like all of life, is filled with uncertainty. The longer I practice medicine, the more I know how little we know. Yet people continue to believe that science will eventually discover the cause or cure of all of their ills. They demand results "yesterday," then cry betrayal when science proceeds slowly. They are surprised when science answers one question only to reveal ten more.

According to Lewis Thomas (109), "The only solid piece of scientific truth about which I feel totally confident is that we are profoundly ignorant about nature. We do not know how humans 'work' or how they 'fit in' to the enormous, imponderable system of life in which we are embedded as working parts." Yet Americans demand answers. Dr. Thomas is concerned that we have become "obsessed with health." Instead of seeking "more exuberance in living, we are busy staving off failure, putting off dying. We are becoming a nation of healthy hypochondriacs, living gingerly, worrying ourselves half to death." He thinks we should worry, most of all, that "our preoccupation with personal health may be a symptom of copping out, an excuse for running upstairs to recline on a couch, sniffing air for contaminants, spraying the room with deodorant, while just outside, the whole of society is coming undone."

So patients with syndromes like fibromyalgia—like Americans in general—need to accept uncertainty. For those of us with chronic illness, the first step to feeling better is to let go of our need for cause; our need to blame someone or something for our illness. Meeting that need does not really help us. In fact, a research study in England found less improvement among patients with CFS who blamed a virus infection than among those who did not rely on this "cause" (110).

The second step is to accept that these syndromes cannot be pigeonholed as physical or mental. They involve complicated interactions of the mind and body. American physicians and society at large tend to regard illness in a dualistic mind *or* body fashion. Since the vast majority of patients with chronic pain, fatigue, sleep and mood disturbances have no obvious structural or physiologic problems, physicians tend to conclude they have a "mental, not a physical problem." Patients often are told, "Well, I can't find anything wrong on your physical examination or your laboratory tests, so I'm going to refer you to a psychiatrist."

Even when illness or disease has a biologic basis, it cannot be explained entirely by genetics or altered chemicals in our brains and bodies. Both patients and health professionals must understand the influence of our childhood, our family, our jobs, and our surroundings on mood and health. Whatever our inborn constitution, it interacts with every aspect of our experiences in shaping our health.

Western medicine has been much slower to embrace these mind-body connections than has Eastern medicine. Actually, in this area, Western medicine has "forgotten" what was embraced by its ancient founders. According to writings attributed to Hippocrates (Epidemics I, ch. 23), each diagnosis must consider human nature, the nature of each individual and the characteristics of each disease.

Physicians should evaluate "physical signs (such as stools, urine, chills, coughing, breathing)" but also "the patient's customs, mode of life, pursuits and age. Then we must consider his speech, his mannerisms, his silences, his thoughts, his habits of sleep or wakefulness and his dreams, their nature and time. Next, we must note whether he plucks his hair, scratches or weeps..."

Mind and body interact not only in the development of illness or disease, but influence how well we fight back or recover. When we first become ill, an infection or other stressor sets in motion a series of reactions in the body (*soma*) and mind (*psyche*). The controversial word *psychosomatic* describes bodily problems that arise in the mind. Used with understanding of mind-body interaction, this is not a demeaning concept!

Medical studies have shown that mood disturbances increase our susceptibility to infection and prolong our recovery from infection. For example, people who developed the Asian flu during the epidemic of 1957 were three times more likely to have pre-existing anxiety and depression than those who did not get this flu (111). Likewise, people with prolonged convalescence from flu and infectious mononucleosis have been more subject to depression and anxiety than those with a shorter convalescence (112).

In what is probably the best study linking our susceptibility of infection to our levels of stress, 394 volunteers were inoculated with various viruses that cause the common cold and upper respiratory infections (113). Following this exposure, subjects who had high levels of recent stress were more likely to develop a significant infection than subjects with lower stress levels.

External or internal stress, from infectious agents to personal crises, causes a series of complicated mind-body reactions. These were first studied extensively by Dr. Hans Selye in the 1950s (114). Our "stress response" is orchestrated by the central nervous system and the immune system (115,116). To give an everyday example, when we trip and almost fall, we feel something in the pit of our stomach. It is a moment of intense physical fear— the same fear we feel when threatened by serious danger. It is created by a cluster of physiologic reactions that include acceleration of our heart and breathing rate. This ancient and automatic "stress response" is designed to give us extra speed and strength to combat danger.

Some stressors are acute, but some are much more persistent, leading to prolonged or repeated stress response. In this case, a maladaptive pattern of hyperarousal may develop. Such hyperarousal can eventually have a negative impact on both the immune system and the central nervous system.

There is bi-directional communication between these systems. The systems and their communication are influenced, in each person, by his or her unique genes, circadian rhythms, and personal experiences. Our stress response is tuned over time by the stress unique to our life. Our personality, coping style, behavior, and emotional state (over time and at the moment of stress) also play a role.

Some aspects of this brain-body connection are hardwired from birth, or even before birth. Sound evidence indicates that the wiring differs between men and women. The female brain responds differently to various stressors than does the male brain. This may help to explain why more women than men suffer fibromyalgia, CFS, migraine, and irritable bowel syndrome.

Like everything else about us, response to stress operates among individuals across a wide "range of normal." In general, however, most responses to stress are dictated by the intensity or duration of stress. They can come and go very fast, though sometimes the response takes awhile to calm down. For example, immune function is suddenly reduced among college students taking important exams or medical students facing their first real patients (117-119). I can relate to that. When presenting my first case—a patient dying of leukemia—to a professor and my fellow medical students, I almost passed out from stress and could not concentrate or sleep well for days afterward.

Of course, among students, stress-reduced immune function is usually a short-term problem. Profound disturbances in immune function are usually the result of prolonged stress. Research found severely lowered immune function among people taking care of relatives with Alzheimer's disease (117,118). Bereavement, such as the death of one's spouse, can have a similar effect. The exact mechanism whereby stress alters immune activity is unclear. Since patients with depression suffer abnormal function of the hypothalamic-pituitary-adrenal axis (HPA axis), depression may be an important key (119). Depression certainly has an adverse impact on the immune system.

The mind-body connection may seem beyond our control but, surprisingly, we can often alter our reaction to stress. One researcher studied laboratory animals who develop an autoimmune disease very similar to lupus (120). Since autoimmune diseases feature an immune response that attacks the self as well as non-self invaders, patients are often treated with medication that curbs the immune system. Such immunosuppressive medication was given to these animals. They were then conditioned—that is, they learned—to associate a drink of sweet fluid with receiving their immune suppressant, cyclophosphamide (Cytoxan). Eventually, receiving the drink alone, without the Cytoxan, had a significant immunosuppressive effect on the animals.

This was one of the first studies to convince scientists that the brain and the nervous system can have a direct influence on the immune system. Such studies have led to the development of the exciting field of psychoneuroimmunology (121). It is now thought that we can each potentially learn ways to modify our own stress response and, through that, our immune response. Rather than automatically reacting to stress in a negative fashion, we can learn techniques to dampen its adverse physiologic effects.

We are only beginning to understand the mind-body interaction, but clearly it exists. It can help us understand chronic illnesses, all of which have mental and physical components. We have already discussed how fear can release epinephrine (adrenaline) and cortisol with resultant increase in our heart rate, blood pressure, and breathing rate. We know that, over time, physical or psychologic stress may trigger or aggravate fibromyalgia, chronic fatigue, insomnia, migraine, low back pain, irritable bowel syndrome and depression (Figure 1) (32).

Our neurohormones and neurotransmitters respond to various stressors in a reproducible fashion. The most promising research related to fibromyalgia and CFS has shown potential for changing the neurohormones of the HPA axis of the brain, as well as neurotransmitters like serotonin and norepinephrine (122). Such research makes intuitive sense since neurotransmitters like serotonin and cortisol control pain sensitivity, muscle energy, fatigue, and how we sleep. They also vary with our levels of stress and our levels of physical activity, which is why exercise is usually good for stress.

Blood flow to areas of the brain is also influenced by these hormones. Compared with healthy control subjects, patients with fibromyalgia have decreased blood flow to the part of the brain that controls pain (81). This may result in a generalized heightened pain perception. In migraine, the blood flow alterations may be very focal, stimulating a release in blood vessel serotonin, which brings on the vascular migraine. Similar research is going on in depression and anxiety disorders.

This new research is exciting and promising, but we must still face uncertainty. It is the X factor in poorly understood illnesses like fibromyalgia. Both physicians and patients must accept more uncertainty to work effectively with these chronic illnesses. Physicians must relent in their search for "disease" and listen more carefully to patients whose symptoms cannot be objectively verified. Patients must relent in their search for causes and cures, and refocus on feeling better.

SECTION IV:
MANAGING
YOUR ILLNESS

Chapter 13:
Finding the right health care providers

The uncertainties of chronic and poorly understood illnesses require a special physician-patient relationship. Patients can easily fall into the trap of "doctor shopping" when frustrated by these illnesses, especially when the diagnosis and treatment plan are in question. But the more confusing the clinical picture, the more important it is to find one physician to trust, who will coordinate the diagnostic evaluation and therapy. This physician, not the patient (my mistake!) should guide the process.

Unfortunately, it isn't easy to find this special relationship. Two trends in modern medicine have placed enormous barriers between patients and their physicians, especially with regard to chronic illness. Ironically, the first barrier is the explosion of scientific technology in the past 20 years. This has enabled great strides in understanding and treating many diseases. However, those very strides may have widened the gap between the art and science of medicine. According to a recent newspaper editorial (123): "The CT and MRI scans, the lasers and the laparoscopies, the chemo-cocktails and DNA codes—all the advances that make modern medicine so effective (and expensive)—have isolated physicians from the patient as a person. In the process, the ancient therapeutic art of listening is being ignored, much to the dismay of many physicians who recognize the limits of technology."

The second threatening trend is the re-organization of medical practice in the United States. What we call "managed-care" may well mismanage people with chronic illness. Such illnesses run counter to cost-cutting measures. They tend to demand expensive health care because they are hard to diagnose and can involve prolonged treatment. They need extra time from the primary physician, just when managed care experts are exerting pressure to shorten office visits. (The "target" at the largest health maintenance organization in New England is for the physician to see 80 patients per week (124). This results in a maximum of 10-15 minutes of time per patient.)

No matter what the medical problem, such pressure results in dissatisfied patients and harried, frustrated physicians. But especially when dealing with chronic illnesses, physicians need time to understand the unique personality and psychosocial issues of each patient. Yet physicians are not reimbursed for the "cognitive" skills involved in lengthy discussion with a family or patient education.

These illnesses are also costly in often requiring a co-ordinated team of care givers. With regard to musculoskeletal pain, the primary care physician may consult with a rheumatologist or physiatrist (a specialist in physical medicine and rehabilitation). Neurologists are helpful in the evaluation and treatment of chronic headaches. Sometimes pain management specialists or sleep treatment specialists are consulted.

Psychiatrists may be called upon to prescribe antidepressant and anti-anxiety medications for patients with major mood disturbances, especially those with poor response to basic medications. Of the many types of mental health therapists, only psychiatrists are medical doctors with the ability to prescribe medication. Primary care physicians can prescribe, but are not always current with the latest psychopharmacology. Nor do they always have the time or training to offer the counseling that should usually accompany medication. Such counseling is best provided by a psychiatrist or some other therapist: psychologist, specially trained social worker, psychiatric clinical nurse specialist, or possibly a religious counselor.

Nowadays, primary care physicians are often penalized for "excess" utilization of consultants. In general, the major incentive under managed care is to "do less." The hardest hit fields are psychiatry and psychology, including the cognitive-behavioral therapy that helped me so much. Most insurers provide little if any coverage for mental health therapy. Patients often have to battle the system to achieve any reasonable long-term mental health treatment. The newer antidepressants have been of great help to patients, but managed health care administrators use their efficacy as ammunition to shoot down requests for long-term psychotherapy (125). They argue that medicines are more effective and less costly than "talk therapy." My opinion, which is widely shared, is that each type of treatment makes the other more effective. Illnesses like fibromyalgia and CFS should be treated with drugs, but also with expert counseling, education, and advice.

Another field hard hit by managed care is physical therapy. It is virtually impossible to receive physical therapy coverage for any illness that is chronic. Likewise, little if any coverage is available for pain management, massage treatments or acupuncture.

The time and cost constraints now imposed upon traditional medicine have pushed dissatisfied patients to seek care elsewhere. Most non-traditional or "alternative" health care providers, including chiropractors and practitioners of homeopathy, are not covered by insurance. Their costs can be considerable if there are repeated visits.

However, they tend to be less expensive per visit. They also tend to spend more time with patients and "touch" them more than most physicians, not only for diagnostic purposes, but as part of the healing process.

With today's focus on biotechnology, the "art of medicine" has become an afterthought to many traditional physicians. Many of us have become less comfortable with our skills in talking to and examining people, and more dependent on the latest technology. This shift threatens a great loss. Those of us who practice traditional medicine could lose the main reason we all chose our profession: to make a difference on a personal level. We would also lose a powerful healing tool: the sense of confidence that we can impart to a patient. Some call this the "placebo effect." As discussed earlier, clinical trials of new drugs compare the medication with placebo, a substance that looks identical but has no medical effect. The medication must test more effective than the placebo. However, in many trials of chronic illness, people receiving placebo are found to improve. Thinking they have received medication, they expect to feel better. They gain confidence that puts mind over matter.

A placebo is not always a pill. Confidence in one's health care providers may elicit a similarly strong response in mind and body. I like to think of this phenomenon as the "karma" established between a physician and patient. We should actively harness this powerful healing tool. More scientific studies should be done to alert physicians to the value of cultivating this art.

One recent study points up the importance of an interactive rather than a passive doctor-patient relationship (126). Patients were asked three questions: Given a treatment choice, would your physician ask you to help make the decision? How often does your physician try to give you some control over your treatment? How often does your physician ask you to take some responsibility for your treatment? Patients were most likely to feel dissatisfied or leave the practice when dealing with physicians who were least interactive.

Particularly patients with chronic illness should seek a physician with an interactive or "participatory" decision-making style. They must work in partnership with their physician. Like all people, physicians vary widely in personality, but you can test their partnership potential by asking yourself these questions:

Do you feel comfortable asking any questions, no matter how absurd they may seem to you? (Incidentally, it can help both of you if you write down your questions before arriving at the office.)

Do you feel rushed during visits? Despite the increased time constraints, some physicians manage to make each patient encounter comprehensive and interactive whereas others do not.

Do you sense a genuine interest in you as a person? Since chronic illnesses involve complicated mind-body and psychosocial interactions, your physician should inquire about your lifestyle, your mood, your family, your support system, and your work.

Of course, you should be sure you have an adequate physical examination followed by informal, personal discussion with the physician. Remember that some degree of physical contact is not only diagnostically important but can be therapeutic.

Be wary of the physician (or any health care provider) who claims to know all the answers. The know-it-all has low participatory potential and may actually know less than practitioners who seem more tentative. In any field, it takes a lot of knowing to know how much you do not know. Certainly in medicine, nobody has all the answers, particularly to questions about chronic illnesses.

Be wary of physicians who order every conceivable test on you, since you may end up having unwarranted procedures. There is a direct association between the number of diagnostic tests ordered and the number of invasive medical and surgical procedures that are performed (127). Be wary also of physicians who send you to every conceivable specialist but may not be listening carefully to you.

Finally, be aware that some very concerned and competent physicians are simply not interested in treating chronic health disorders. They prefer a different type of challenge. They may dutifully exclude all "serious" illness and then say: "You'll just have to learn to live with your headaches" or your back pain, fibromyalgia, chronic fatigue, etc. They are only half-right. Patients do indeed need to learn how to accept uncertainty and live with these illnesses, as this book has stressed. However, the learning process should be guided by a health professional. Patients should not be turned loose to manage alone. Those of us who suffer chronic illness need a physician to share with us the responsibility for getting better—a physician who is interested in chronic illnesses.

In cooperating as partners, the patient and physician must work toward a balance. Patients can balance feelings of helplessness by taking some measure of control and participating in decision-making, but this forces physicians to find a balance too. In any partnership, sharing control and decision-making usually takes practice and trust. Traditionally, physicians have taken a paternal approach to patients. Many fear that patients lack the medical knowledge and perhaps the strength or good sense (especially when sick or in pain) to make good decisions. They feel responsible for patients and do not want to shirk responsibility by giving leeway that may result in a bad decision. However, recent studies indicate these concerns may be exaggerated. Physicians treating chronic pain have tended to give narcotics very sparingly for fear of addicting patients. Many have resisted giving patients control of their own dose, as with a morphine "pump." Yet studies show that patients using such pumps actually use *less narcotic* than when pre-set doses are given them, at set intervals, by a physician or nurse.

As patients with chronic illness work with their physician, they should gather information from other sources. Here again, balance is important. Ask your health care team for sources of information and outside reading, and attend educational seminars—but avoid preoccupation with the search. Do not neglect your other life interests. Do not let the barriers of your illness interfere more than they must. Keep trying, and you may find you can leap over some of those obstacles.

Finally, you will need to relinquish some control of your health to your health care providers. You also need to ask and accept support from family and friends. Do as much as you can, but be flexible when you are not feeling well. My own style, in work and life in general, was always to push ahead, to go full-force toward my goals. As I would with any other project, I initially threw all my energy into "curing" my illnesses. Such energy is good, but not when it represents a need for control (or the appearance of control). Needing to feel in control of my illness and "leaving no stone unturned" in looking for a cure brought me nothing but preoccupation, frustration, anger, and exhaustion.

Once I accepted the limitations of not being able to control all aspects of my health, I was much better off. I began to feel better and enjoy more of what mattered in my life.

Chapter 14:
Medications

The large number of medications used to treat chronic pain, fatigue, sleep and mood disorders points to the sad fact that none of them is highly effective. However, many have some value and patients should be familiar with what they can and cannot do.

Pain medications come in two main categories. There are simple or non-specific analgesics (pain relievers) like acetaminophen (e.g., Tylenol) or codeine. Then there are analgesics that also combat inflammation. For example, a few aspirin a day is analgesic whereas 12 a day may be anti-inflammatory. The simple analgesics block pain receptors in the nervous system but have no direct effect on the "cause" of pain. The more potent are often habit-forming narcotics, and physicians usually resist prescribing them for chronic pain. However, some specialists in the treatment of pain argue that narcotics can be used with little fear of addiction, provided careful monitoring is in place. Meanwhile, we now have more potent non-narcotic pain relievers, such as Ultram, now being tested in the treatment of fibromyalgia and chronic low back pain.

The anti-inflammatory analgesics not only relieve pain but chemically block the inflammation process. They include the corticosteroids, such as prednisone, and the nonsteroidal anti-inflammatory medications (NSAIDS, or "en-seds") like ibuprofen, naproxen, and aspirin (Table 8). Anti-inflammatory medications are best used for the pain of diseases like rheumatoid arthritis that involve inflammation of joints, muscles, or other tissues. The illnesses we are discussing rarely involve inflammation, so steroids and NSAIDS are used mainly for pain relief. Steroids have much toxicity and little efficacy as pain relievers, but NSAIDS can be helpful at very low doses. Low doses of ibuprofen or naproxen can "take the edge off pain" and are quite safe, though with long-term use must be watched for gastrointestinal or kidney problems. Tylenol is generally safer and may be just as helpful.

Many patients find Tylenol or aspirin quite sufficient. They are often surprised to hear that aspirin is an NSAID, working against inflammation as well as pain. It really is quite a miracle drug, a surprisingly strong medication in view of its negligible side effects and cost. It can irritate the stomach, possibly more than newer NSAIDS. Prescription is "empirical," or trial and error, since response is highly individual. A physician might recommend 4-6 aspirin or Tylenol daily for these illnesses.

Medications to suppress or enhance the immune system, are in general not helpful and not prescribed for the chronic illnesses we are discussing. Despite those who blame the immune system (or a virus) for disorders like fibromyalgia and CFS, no evidence has yet been found.

Medications to treat migraine also come in two types: those that prevent attacks and those that abort an attack that has already begun (Table 8). Examples of preventive migraine medicines include the beta blockers, such as propanolol; calcium channel blockers, such as verapamil; and

the old standby, tricyclic antidepressants, such as amitriptyline. Sumatriptan (Imitrex) appears to be the most effective medicine yet formulated to abort an attack of migraine before it becomes full-blown. Other medications
used to abort a migraine headache include NSAIDS, steroids, various narcotic analgesics and the ergot derivatives, such as Cafergot. Ergot is a fungus that infects rye
plants. Its effects on the human nervous system can be
helpful or harmful, depending on how it is administered.

Since the syndromes discussed in this book share
many overlapping features, it's no surprise that they share
medications. In particular, low doses of the anti-depressants have proven widely helpful, not only with mood
disturbances but with the pain and sleep problems of
fibromyalgia and CFS. This makes sense in view of the
action of neurohormones on pain, sleep, and blood-flow
to the brain. As mentioned earlier, antidepressants like
Prozac, have also been effective for women with PMS
(101).

However, the choice of medications will vary with
each patient. It depends on which symptoms are the most
prominent, the duration of the illness, the patient's age,
the various side effects, and physician experience and
preference. Some patients are highly sensitive to the side-
effects of many medications.

In selecting medications, one of the first factors to consider is the presence or absence of major depression or
anxiety. Among patients with chronic illness or disease,
25-50 percent suffer depression and anxiety, which can
and should be treated. As noted earlier, untreated depression not only adds suffering: it can hinder adaptation to
illness, slow recovery, and raise the risk of recurrence.
Fortunately, the last decade has seen a virtual explosion
of effective medications to treat depression and anxiety
(Table 9). At least two-thirds of people respond very well
to antidepressant medications. As we know more about

the biologic basis for depression, anxiety, and other mood disturbances, more effective medicines have been developed. Each affects neurotransmitters in the central nervous system, such as serotonin and neuroadrenaline.

The older tricyclic antidepressants like Elavil and the newer agents like Prozac are equally effective in the treatment of depression. However, the newer agents tend to have fewer side effects (Table 9). Those especially well-tolerated by patients include the new serotonin reuptake inhibitors like fluoxetine (Prozac), paroxetine (Zoloft), sertraline (Paxil) and other new agents such as nefazodone (Serzone). People who do not respond to these can often benefit from monoamine oxidase inhibitors (MAOs), but these medications impose various dietary restrictions.

In fibromyalgia, CFS, and their associated illnesses, medications must usually be selected and tuned to each individual by a process of trial and error. It is impossible to tell who will respond to what. If pain predominates, I usually begin with a low dose of a tricyclic antidepressant at nighttime and simple analgesics during the day. These mild drugs, with their minimal side effects, are often sufficient. But if fatigue is more troublesome, I may first use a serotonin reuptake inhibitor, taken in the morning. (Night-time use of such medications can actually keep people awake.) If clinical depression is not present, I prescribe these antidepressants at much lower doses than usually prescribed to treat depression.

Side effects can often be minimized by a combination of medications, each given at a low dose (if depression is not present). A patient might take a low morning dose of one of the newer serotonin reuptake inhibitors, such as 10 mgs of Prozac or 50 mgs of Zoloft, combined with a low night-time dose of tricyclic antidepressant, such as 10-25 mgs of Elavil (17). Tricyclic medications have been found to be effective in a number of chronic pain conditions, including fibromyalgia (16), low back pain (128) and non-cardiac chest pain (129). The newer medications, such as Prozac, seem more useful for battling fatigue. They can also help people to cope better with their chronic illness.

As scientists understand better the mysterious pain pathways involved in chronic illness, more "targeted" drugs will be available. Such medications will interact very specifically with a tiny target—and only that target—in the central nervous system. This means they will more effectively relieve pain and, at the same time, cause fewer side effects. As we know more about the relevant neuro-hormones and neurotransmitters, drugs that alter these compounds will be tested in fibromyalgia, CFS, and related diseases. We can be very hopeful, although the complexity of these illnesses makes it unlikely that we can find a "silver bullet." We will continue to sort through many treatments and medications, by trial and error, but our choices and outcomes will steadily improve.

Chapter 15:
Exercise and Physical Methods to Combat Pain

In combination with medication, a gentle program of cardiovascular fitness can greatly benefit most patients with fibromyalgia, chronic fatigue syndrome, chronic low back pain, sleep disturbances and depression. Often, patients who enjoyed exercise before becoming ill have stopped all kinds of activity from pain, fatigue, or fear that activity will make them worse. However, they usually find that the right approach to exercise makes them feel better.

Any exercise program should be carefully tailored to the patient's age and previous level of physical activity. It should be started at a low level and gradually increased. Perhaps most important, it must blend and balance periods of activity with periods of rest.

Cardiovascular exercise may sound daunting, but it simply involves activity that slightly increases your heart-rate for a period of time. It might include brisk walking outdoors or on a treadmill, biking, swimming or other water exercises, such as water aerobics or water jogging. Patients should work up to a minimum of 30 minutes, at least 3 times per week. The exercise should increase your heart-rate to within its "target zone." This zone lies within

60-80 percent of your target heart-rate, which you calculate by subtracting your age from 220. If you are 50, your target heart-rate is 170. Your target zone is 60-80 percent of 170, or 100 to 130 beats per minute. When exercising within this zone, you should feel slightly breathless but still able to maintain a conversation. Whatever activity you enjoy, be sure to warm up and cool down for a few minutes. A few stretches before and after exercise are increasingly important as we get older.

Cardiovascular exercise is not only good for general fitness. It has been shown to raise our spirits and actually to have a pain-relieving effect at high levels of intensity. Intense exercise releases endorphins from the brain that can kill pain better than morphine. These "natural opiates" probably explain why athletes can perform in spite of injury without feeling much pain. Cardiovascular exercise has also been demonstrated to improve immune function and to lessen the chance of getting infections. To achieve such benefits requires more exertion than is generally recommended for patients with chronic illness. However, even modest exercise, if combined with relaxation techniques, can definitely reduce pain and increase your energy level. Studies suggest that the optimal time to exercise is in the late afternoon or early evening, but whatever fits into your schedule will do.

Millions of people in China, including the elderly, have been doing tai-chi and chi-gong every morning for centuries. Such ancient arts, including yoga from India, have become increasingly popular in the U.S. Although yoga is most well known for its meditative state, its active forms involve very useful stretching and strengthening. Any form of exercise that makes our bodies move and quiets our minds at the same time is worth doing. Stretching and exercises to improve flexibility will ease chronic muscle spasms. We use yoga in the stress-reduction and mindfulness segment of our pain management program.

Most patients with arthritis and fibromyalgia have found it very helpful.

The stretches of yoga or other approaches to exercise should generally be practiced at first with the help of a teacher to ensure safety and proper technique. Training and monitoring is even more important when patients try resistance exercises like "nautilus" or "free weights." Since "bulking up" is not the goal, we recommend more repetitions with minimal weight resistance. Modest weight training exercise is beneficial because it can decrease the risk of heart disease as well as improving joints, coordination, and general quality of life. Stretching, strengthening, and cardiovascular fitness exercises have proven beneficial even when started by people aged 75 to 85. The same seems to apply with resistance exercise. These forms of exercise appear to complement each other. One study found that a weight-training program improved the walking endurance of healthy elderly people (130). There are no age limits to modest cardiovascular or weight-training exercise.

Other methods to combat pain include such "hands on" treatment as traditional physical therapy, massage, and manipulation. Some types are passive: you sit and relax while the therapist is massaging, manipulating, or probing. Alternatively, a machine like ultrasound or electrical stimulation ("E-stim" or TENS) is applied. Other methods are more active and require that therapist and patient work together.

Tender point and trigger point injections using a local anesthetic such as lidocaine can be effective. They especially help with regional myofascial pain, muscular headaches, and chronic back pain. They may also help with fibromyalgia and CFS, but so far we have not proven this with scientific studies. Injections are usually done at the site of maximum muscle tenderness and spasm. They are much safer than corticosteroid injections, which can have local and systemic side effects.

Patients with fibromyalgia do not generally benefit from corticosteroid injections. However, if inflammation is present (like bursitis or tendinitis), steroid injections may be used. In treating back pain, epidural steroid injections are sometimes helpful.

Some of my patients have benefited from acupuncture and acupressure, as well as techniques such as myofascial release. The role of such modalities in treating many illnesses is being explored. Acupuncture in particular seems promising for fibromyalgia since the typical acupuncture locations largely coincide with the tender and trigger points. The clinical importance of these tender points and trigger points is "news" to Western medicine, but has long been known to Eastern medicine.

I generally advise my patients with fibromyalgia, CFS and related illnesses that we want to try a number of different physical modalities to combat their pain. We want to interrupt the vicious cycle of pain leading to muscle spasm, leading to diminished blood supply, leading to more pain. Whether a treatment works more locally (such as a massage or trigger point injections) or more systemically (such as cardiovascular exercise or biofeedback) is immaterial as long as it helps.

Once patients are started on a combination of medication and physical activity, they need to take another step on their own. Anyone with a chronic degree of muscle pain and spasm is more prone to the everyday muscle strains and injuries that happen to everyone. Patients already in pain from chronic illness certainly do not want to bring on more pain! So they need to take more responsibility for how they move. They must become more careful and pay more attention to how they work, exercise, or simply pick up a child. Patients need to develop proper "ergonomics", i.e. better ways to move through their daily activities. This can be a simple matter of bending the knees when lifting objects from a low position, or using a chair with back support. It can be complicated, especially if your work routine requires a lot of repetitive motion. In those situations, I may ask an occupational therapist or work rehabilitation specialist to explore the work environment and help the patient develop better techniques and habits. Either way, with or without such help, patients need to concentrate and learn new moves that may not "come naturally."

Like other aspects of treatment, exercise must be conducted with a sense of balance. I had always persuaded myself that exercise would take care of any stress that I had. In fact, I was addicted to exercise. Often, the most obsessive-compulsive exercise enthusiasts have a pathologic preoccupation with body image or a history of some eating disorder, such as anorexia or bulimia. For most of my life, exercise was an obsession; if I went a single day without my usual intense work-out, I felt tired and blue. However, all the fun from exercise that I knew as a boy had long since evaporated. I would push through the exercise routine like a robot, not knowing exactly what I was doing or why I was doing it.

This excess exercise, which I saw also in many friends and patients, was suddenly brought home to me in a movie called *That's Life*. In one scene, a character played by Jack Lemmon is facing his 60th birthday. Totally consumed with his imagined ills and mortality, he is oblivious to a very real medical crisis that threatens his wife, played by Julie Andrews. One morning at 3 a.m., Andrews wakes to find Lemmon in a frenzy, biking as fast as possible on his stationary bike while constantly checking his heart-rate with a stethoscope. She asks what on earth he is doing and, in his feverish fog of exercise, Lemmon says he is trying to "bicycle myself to death."

I've tried to change my ways and avoid the extreme portrayed by Jack Lemmon. Sometimes when I am exercising at the health club, I see that frenzied look on the faces of people trying desperately to exercise away their pain and suffering. Like everything else that is "good for you," exercise can also be bad for you. I often see people exercising "through the pain," causing muscles and joints further injury. Too much exercise at too great a pace can even affect the immune response and other systems, as when it curtails menstruation, leading to bone loss, in some female athletes.

Nowadays I purposely do not exercise vigorously every day. Evidence suggests that the body needs to rest a day between intense bouts. So I take the day off or do something gentle, such as stretches or some yoga for 30 minutes. When I do exercise, I try to avoid feeling competitive with everyone around me. I have learned to be happy with less lofty goals. Now that I exercise with a sense of balance and moderation, I am enjoying it more.

Chapter 16:
Non-traditional treatment

N on-traditional or alternative medicine includes a growing range of old and new health interventions that lie outside the Western tradition of medicine. Such interventions are not necessarily invalid or harmful—in fact, some are very useful. But very few have ever been scientifically tested. Their safety and efficacy are largely "unproven." They frequently cannot even be defined with consistency.

Alternative treatments are best considered as complementary to traditional medical management. They understandably attract patients with chronic illness and other problems that are poorly understood and not readily cured by the medical establishment. A recent survey found that one-third of all Americans used at least one form of "unconventional" therapy (3). This included chiropractic treatment, relaxation techniques, massage, imagery, acupuncture, spiritual healing, life-style diets, herbal medicine, megavitamins, energy healing, and homeopathy.

Such treatments were sought largely for the common illnesses covered in this book. Patients often combined them with visits to a traditional physician, but rarely mentioned their unconventional care. This unfortunate finding suggests they did not feel they could be open with their physician. They were not working as partners, and the physician had no chance to advise them on therapies that might be risky. The safest therapy—conventional or unconventional—can be risky when it is inadvertantly mixed with others because a physician is prescribing in the dark. To avoid dangerous clashes of therapy, any care giver needs to know a patient's total care picture.

The scientists who conducted the survey reported that, in 1990, Americans made an estimated 425 million visits to nontraditional practitioners—far more than their visits to primary care physicians (3). Their unconventional treatments cost an estimated $13.7 billion, of which three-quarters was paid out of pocket. In this day and age of high medical costs, it is amazing to see how much patients are spending on common, chronic disorders like fibromyalgia, headache and back pain—and on therapies that are totally unproven.

Patients appear to be turning to such treatments more and more. Alternative therapy was used by 91% of fibromyalgia patients and 63% of those with other musculoskeletal disorders (131). Seventy percent of the fibromyalgia patients used alternative products such as herbs and lotions, 48% used spiritual practices, 40% saw alternative practitioners, and 26% tried dietary modifications (Table 10). Patient satisfaction was highest with spiritual practices, including prayer and meditation, and with alternative practitioners. Of the latter, patients were most satisfied with chiropractors, massage therapists, and acupuncturists.

We are in an age where non-conventional medical approaches are becoming mainstream rather than "alternative." Many of them loosely represent the venerable "holistic" philosophy. This teaches that human beings, like any organism, must be treated as a whole. Mind and body do not operate independently but are blended in the organism, which is more than the sum of its parts.

Holistic medicine is an old idea that is regaining popularity for many reasons. A primary reason may be the failure of modern traditional medicine to explain the mechanisms of many common and chronic illnesses. Another may be the growing gap between the art and science of medicine, which can make the medical profession seem impersonal. Some overzealous and even unscrupulous practitioners have jumped on the holistic bandwagon. This is especially unfortunate since holistic and traditional medicine need not be adversaries. John Sarno recently wrote: "Perhaps holistic should be defined as that which includes consideration of both the emotional and structural aspects of health and illness. In accepting this definition one does not reject the scientific method. All physicians should be practitioners of 'holistic medicine' in the sense that they recognize the interaction between mind and body. *To leave the emotional dimension out of the study of health and illness is poor medicine and poor science"*(132). The italics are mine.

However, non-traditional medicine has claimed to be more holistic than traditional medicine. It seems more natural because of its focus on natural remedies, often derived from plants or our own hormones. Many such "non-traditional" treatments are traditional to Eastern medicine. Herbs and other natural medications have been used for centuries in China. Even in the West, some of our most important drugs are "herbals" with a very long history. One is digitalis, the heart medication derived from the foxglove plant. Another is the ancient analgesic and anti-inflammatory drug derived from willow bark: salicylic acid, or aspirin.

Eastern medicine emphasizes the maintenance of a balance in life and health. For the Chinese, chi represents the harmony of life forces in and around us. Illness arises when the natural flow of these forces is misdirected. To restore harmony, Eastern medicine has relied much less on synthetically-manufactured drugs than on the healing power we can derive from nature or from ourselves. It has much to teach Western medicine and Western people. However, the "holistic" care now pushed at us is often a far cry from the Eastern philosophy of serene moderation. Alternative medicine has spawned a multi-million dollar industry in the United States. The public is inundated with all kinds of folk remedies, health foods and vitamins. We are bombarded with unproven methods of psychic and physical healings that are said to cure everything from aging to the common cold.

The claims and choices are mind-boggling. One has to consider that some alternative practitioners are less interested in healing than in making a quick buck. The more promises we hear, the more we should beware. Browsing recently through a book store in Boston, I counted 25 books on nutrition and our health, 20 on the mind-body connection, 15 on depression, 12 on chronic back pain, 8 on the chronic fatigue syndrome, 6 on the "yeast connection," 5 on headaches, 4 on irritable bowel syndrome, and 3 on chronic muscle pain, including fibromyalgia. Many of these books contained a series of health formulas and step-wise approaches "destined" to lead the reader to better health. Some are based on good sense and good ideas, but many are not.

What might be called "naturopathy" often promotes some natural substance said to alleviate many of our common ills. This substance is often a display centerpiece of health food stores. The current favorite is melatonin, a hormone secreted from the pineal gland in our brain. It promotes sleep and may become an important treatment for jet lag and other disturbances of sleep or circadian rhythm. Though undeniably "natural," melatonin has not been adequately tested to prove its real capabilities. Nor do we know its potential toxicities when used over months or years.

Natural substances are not always truly natural, nor always benign. After all, many poisons are natural, and our own body can attack us. Some substances promoted as "natural" are synthetically manufactured or come from the glands of other animals, not humans. This alone does not make them bad, but in the famous case of L-trypto-phan, the manufacturing process caused a dangerous impurity. L-tryptophan was the melatonin of the 1980s, with claims to help sleep, mood, and energy. However, it was found to cause adverse reactions and occasionally the life-threatening "eosinophilia-myalgia syndrome."

Some people shun prescription medicines as "unnat-ural," even though FDA approved manufacturing pro-cedures are designed to ensure safety and uniformity. They worry about side effects listed on the label, yet these too are evidence of safety regulation. When "natural" medications do not list side effects, this does not mean they have none! We simply have no clue.

Natural or unnatural, any substance that can do good in the human body can also do harm, if only in rare indi-viduals under rare circumstances. In traditional or non-traditional medicine, what we look for is the substance or therapy that does the most good for the most people, most of the time, with the fewest side effects.

We must often settle for a trade-off. This applies not only to medications but to human hormones used in treat-ment. Hormones might be seen as the most "natural" of therapies, but they have their toxicities and side effects. Corticosteroids, a hormone derived from the adrenal gland, is the most potent antiinflammatory and immu-nosuppressive medication we have today. When first dis-covered, it was hailed as a miracle—and it can be when treating a disease like asthma or lupus. However, we soon discovered its serious side-effects and now avoid its pro-longed use at high dose, except to treat highly threatening disease.

Another miracle hormone is estrogen. Its natural secretion drops with menopause, but estrogen replacement therapy can reduce the risk of heart disease and osteoporosis in postmenopausal women. Recent studies suggest it may even reduce the risk of Alzheimer's disease. Estrogen is often used short-term to alleviate hot flashes, sleep disturbances and mood disturbances associated with menopause or PMS. However, in some women, estrogens have unpleasant side effects. Studies also suggest that they raise the risk of certain cancers to a small but significant degree. Thus benefits of this hormone must be weighed against its possible adverse effects.

Several hormones related to steroids and manufactured by the adrenal glands may prove beneficial in treating chronic illness. Two that have caught the public eye are growth hormone and dehydroepiandrosterone or DHEA. Their role in medicine is not yet clear. However, since their levels decline as we age, it seems logical that raising those levels could help the body age better. Researchers found a low level of growth hormone in one-third of patients with fibromyalgia. Their pain was reduced when growth hormone was supplied (22). This is exciting news, but we do not know how helpful such treatment might be. Furthermore, growth hormone currently must be administered by daily injection at a cost of $800-1000 per month. DHEA is being evaluated for the treatment of lupus and other immunologic connective tissue diseases. It is felt by some to be useful in treating conditions like fibromyalgia, but more research evidence is needed. Yet, you can walk into any pharmacy or many fitness centers and purchase DHEA and melatonin.

These and other "natural" substances may prove helpful in the treatment of chronic illness. But they should not be promoted or prescribed until scientific studies establish their safety and efficacy. Such studies are the ticket to mainstream medicine. As noted above, the advantage of prescription medication is the very intense review process it goes through to get FDA approval. Without that approval, most drugs cannot be legally used in this country. They cannot be sold without a listing of side effects, no matter how rare and unlikely they are. Products like DHEA and melatonin have bypassed FDA approval because they are not classified as drugs.

Unfortunately, some patients become so concerned about potential side-effects of prescribed medicines that they stop taking them before getting any benefit! They do not wait to find out if the drug will help them. In fact, they may do themselves harm by stopping a drug too soon. Most antibiotics, for example, need time to kill all the bacteria; with insufficient time, they kill only the weakest, leaving the worst to cause a relapse.

In time, many products touted by non-traditional health care providers will undoubtedly be rejected as worthless. However, traditional medicine must be open-minded enough to recognize that some deserve a place in the mainstream. Certain nutritional and homeopathic products may be likely candidates. Homeopathy is a form of medicine that treats disease with drugs capable of producing in healthy persons the symptoms of the disease to be treated. Homeopathic drugs are given in such minute amounts that they probably have little effect (good or bad) so the patient simply gets well. In times when traditional physicians relied on bleeding, purging, and other drastic measures, homeopathy at least "did not harm." Several respected hospitals still carry on the name (if not wholly the philosophy) of Samual Hahnemann, the 19th century founder of homeopathy. Most modern physicians take an "allopathic" approach and are skeptical about homeopathy. Nevertheless, some medications that we commonly use in conventional medicine were first used in homeopathic medicine. These include nitroglycerin, a mainstay of treatment for angina, and gold, used to treat rheumatoid arthritis. A few controlled, scientific studies have found some improvement from homeopathic treatment of people with fibromyalgia (133), osteoarthritis (134), and rheumatoid arthritis (135).

All these natural approaches to health are currently very popular in the United States. So far, few are known to cause ill effects. But many cause zero effects (at considerable cost) and divert people from traditional therapies proven to be helpful. We have seen toxicities, as in the case of L-tryptophan. We know that certain Chinese herbal medicines can cause serious liver and kidney disease (136,137). Macrobiotic and cult diets have been associated with severe malnutrition and other problems (138,139). The whole area of "naturopathy" needs much more scientific investigation.

Chiropractic therapy and acupuncture have been subjected to some recent well-done studies. They have shown real benefit and are increasingly accepted by the medical establishment. Actually, many chiropractors do not consider themselves "alternative" practitioners. The general consensus, in traditional medicine, is that chiropractic care can be helpful in the treatment of back pain and other musculoskeleletal problems. A recent study showed chiropractic and conventional medicine to produce similar outcomes for patients with acute low back pain (140). Chiropractic treatment was associated with increased patient satisfaction but also with increased costs. Acupuncture has shown some utility in the treatment of rheumatoid arthritis (141) and osteoarthritis (142).

Holistic medicine contributes most importantly to traditional medicine by fostering more appreciation of the connection of our physical and emotional well-being. It has developed techniques to bridge the perceived gap between mind and body. Physicians and patients need to know how to blend physical and meditational approaches to illness, and when to shift from one to the other. Some patients benefit most from physical modalities such as ultrasound, electrical stimulation of tense muscles, or types of manipulation therapy. Others benefit more from meditative approaches like individual or group therapy, yoga, meditation or prayer.

Above all, the goal of holistic or other therapies should be to give patients more independence and control in dealing with their illness. The more dependency that any treatment fosters, the more it is likely to fail in the long run. For this reason, successful holistic practitioners in New England, such as Jon Kabat-Zinn and Herbert Benson, offer self-help programs to complement treatment of many chronic illnesses (53,143). The courses go beyond the physician-patient relationship, which by its nature can foster dependency. They lead people to learn for themselves. Courses usually involve an intensive ten- or twelve-week program of weekly sessions where participants explore mindfulness, meditation, gentle stretching and yoga or tai-chi.

In my own practice, we offer a similar program to explore the role of stress and its impact on illness. We try to change patients' unrealistic fears or expectations. We encourage them to follow the program with self-directed use of techniques they found most beneficial: meditation or yoga or just quiet sitting. Ideally, such techniques will become an ingrained part of their lives. Just as one must regularly exercise to maintain physical conditioning, one must pursue mind-body practices with continuity. Many patients find that self-help groups cheer them along and keep them on track. Such groups can be very important in the promotion of wellness and independence. However, I believe that some professional advice and guidance should be maintained. Patients who feel improved need not see their care giver as often, but if they come in only "as needed," they may wait too long. They may come in when they have already lost ground that will be hard to regain.

As I worked with my own illnesses, a combination of medication and stress reduction were most important in helping me think clearly about my pain and stress. At first I found this thinking very difficult, as do many of my patients. They often say, "I don't want to think about my pain at all. I want to forget it. I want it to go away. I want to be the way that I was." Distraction from pain and stress may seem helpful, but it only goes so far. We still have to accept that we are in pain and under stress. We still have to accept the uncertainty of chronic illness and recognize that much of what we feel is an emotional reaction to our illness. However difficult our core symptoms, we can at least tone down our reaction to them. We can alleviate this additional suffering if we will face the role we play in it.

Finding peace and calm during the storm of illness and uncertainty can be helpful to anyone. The search takes commitment and practice. Although I am still a novice at meditation and yoga, I do feel physical and emotional peace and greater balance when I truly concentrate on these relaxation techniques. For many of my patients with fibromyalgia, CFS, and chronic pain, these techniques have brought relief from illness and proven helpful in life as a whole.

Chapter 17:
Ten steps to living better with chronic illness

1) Accepting uncertainty in our illness is necessary before we can begin to feel better.

Most human beings want to be able to control their lives. Particularly in our society, we have the idea that life's events are produced by specific conditions. We seek causes, certainty, and predictability. Western science and medicine share these values and seem to promise solutions to problems like chronic illness. If solutions come slowly or bring new problems, we blame science. If no one can tell us exactly how to get better, we blame our physicians. But in most chronic illnesses like fibromyalgia and CFS, we are living with uncertainty every day of our lives.

We need to accept not having all the answers regarding our health. There are no physical findings, blood tests, or X-ray abnormalities that are clearly associated with fibromyalgia, chronic fatigue syndrome, chronic low back pain, irritable bowel syndrome, migraine or depression. Thus we must accept inexact diagnoses—or no diagnoses at all, since some physicians are not familiar with these illnesses or, more often, do not accept them as specific medical entities. Seeking diagnosis, many people then seek multiple opinions and treatments, some of which may be at odds. When finally diagnosed with one of these illnesses, many patients don't feel very relieved. After all, they still face treatment uncertainty. They still wonder if and when the problems will ever go away.

The fact is that medicine does not have all the answers, especially with regard to these illnesses. No practitioner, no matter how informed or well-meaning, can tell you how they will affect your life. Some of this affect is in your hands. Struggling with uncertainty can, in itself, cause chaos and misery in our lives and health. If you can give up some of the struggle—the part that does no good— you will be ready for the next step: letting go.

2) You can not control your illness but can modify its impact on your life by letting go of unrealistic expectations.

It is natural to wonder what will happen next in an illness, to worry that it might get worse, to look for ways to make it better. With conditions like a heart attack, physicians can offer predictions and suggestions. The better a disease is understood, the easier it is for them to tell people how they can positively affect their disease. For example, high blood pressure, or hypertension, is a major risk factor for a heart attack. We can often lower this risk if we take medication and stop smoking, lose weight, and increase our physical exercise. However, with chronic illness such as fibromyalgia, chronic fatigue syndrome, migraine, and irritable bowel syndrome, physicians do not know the risk factors. They cannot tell people how to prevent or modify these illnesses. Certain medications and other therapies can help, but must be used by trial and error. Treatments may not work, and they never cure—though the illness may eventually go away.

The trick is to "let go" without giving up. "Letting go" does not mean "giving up" or taking a fatalistic outlook.

It means recognizing that we cannot totally control our health any more than we can totally control our lives. Bad things may happen to us that are beyond our control. The good news is that people are amazingly resilient and can usually bounce back from the gravest misfortune—if they truly want to.

In my own case, letting go seemed the last thing I needed to do. I wanted to grab my health and make it behave! As I floundered in a sea of uncertain diagnoses, treatment, and prognosis, I kept asking myself: "What could I have done to prevent this illness? What can I now do differently to make it go away?" But I could find no answers, and once I let go of this fruitless search—and blaming myself—I became more flexible in adapting to my illness.

Letting go requires concentration. This requires calming the mind, one of the most difficult meditation techniques to learn. Of course, calming the mind is especially difficult during times of stress, illness, and worry about one's health and future—just when we need calming the most! But with practice, we can turn our minds from the racing and unrealistic thoughts that make us more anxious.

3) Lacking total control of our illness does not mean we have NO control.

One obvious "symptom" that we can control is our stress response. The more we can keep ourselves grounded and not let our minds run away with us, the better. Counseling, psychotherapy, cognitive therapy, meditation, and yoga can all help us to stay focused, to take things moment by moment.

We can't modify the inherited or genetic factors that affect our illness or our stress response. But we can adapt and change other factors. We can strengthen our body with exercise, broaden our mind with education and counseling, modify our diet, our job, and our life satisfaction. We should play an active role in these illness factors that we can change. But we must always bear in mind that some factors remain beyond our control.

Taking these positive steps is difficult if your health care providers have given you unrealistic expectations. They can be unrealistically negative, as when a physician says "nothing can be done." They can be unrealistically positive, as when alternative practitioners say illness can be banished by some kind of "positive thinking." Positive thinking is always helpful, but people feel guilty when they "fail" to cure themselves. They blame themselves when they cannot "control" or will away their illness.

In general, false hopes and cures are detrimental when we are afflicted with a chronic illness. We must let them go, along with self-blame. We need to give up the inclination to blame someone or something else for our illness. Our mechanistic belief that our health is always determined by specific factors, within or outside of us, does not work for chronic illnesses.

4) Find the right health care "partner" to direct your care.

You need to find a practitioner who can coordinate the management of your illness. I naturally favor a physician, given our comprehensive training and access to various modalities. Whether family practitioner, internist, rheumatologist or alternative practitioner, this care giver must above all accept disorders like fibromyalgia as discrete and important illnesses. He or she must be a good listener, open to your thoughts and suggestions, willing to consult with appropriate specialists and to coordinate a team approach. If this coordinator is a traditional physician, he or she should be open to trying innovative and alternative treatments if traditional medical management is not working.

5) Explore the mind and body connection and learn how to manage it.

Stress, whether physical or emotional, is very important in chronic illness. You must learn ways to handle it better and be open to assistance. Medications can help. Those that affect the brain are often more effective than those that affect the rest of the body. Try to accept this fact without feeling that your illness is "all in your head." The fact is that 30-50% of patients with fibromyalgia and CFS, as well as migraine and low back pain, are also suffering from significant depression and anxiety.

These are not "weaknesses" but legitimate disorders. Whether they are part of your reaction to illness or part of a biologic predisposition, they must be treated. They represent a part of your illness that can be alleviated. Usually people take these medications short-term to "get back on their feet." It is tragic that, despite all we are learning about brain chemistry, too many Americans still avoid taking anti-depressant and anti-anxiety medications. They feel a stigma or have unreasonable fears. They imagine they should be able to "pull themselves together" or let depression "run its course." But even if they could, why turn away from a safe medication that can help? If we accept medication for physical pain, why not for mental pain? Untreated mental pain is a risk factor for many other problems.

6) Use every source to gain knowledge about your illness, but check what you learn with your care coordinator.

I encourage patients to learn about their illness but always worry that they may be unduly influenced by "the gospel according to X authority." No one source has all the answers about chronic illness. Perspective is important. Patients must remember that certain physicians, alternative practitioners and support groups tend to promote a biased account of research findings. The media may choose to focus on the most exciting but unproven claims. The "Internet" offers endless information that is rarely "filtered" through scientific or medically sophisticated channels. Patients should bounce whatever they learn off their health care coordinator to make sure their information is balanced and objective. To paraphrase the old saying, "A little learning is a dangerous thing." A little information, especially if biased, can block patients from gathering the many facts and ideas that will make them truly informed.

7) Look beyond the label of your illness to focus on the overlapping features of related syndromes.

The illnesses we have been exploring are poorly understood but widely accepted to be overlapping syndromes that make people ill (Figure 3). Science needs to keep searching for better definitions—not to mention cause and cure!—but patients should not worry about the current labels. In general and in each individual case, the common nature of these illnesses is what matters. It is not important to know whether you have fibromyalgia or CFS or both unless the treatment would vary, based on a specific diagnosis. Currently, the treatment is very similar for each of these chronic illnesses.

8) Be flexible: try new approaches to your illness and life in general. Your adaptation to illness can actually help you grow as a person.

Many patients have told me that their illness made them a stronger and happier person. This is certainly true in my own case. I now feel more at peace with myself. Meeting the challenge and uncertainty of physical and psychological pain has forced me to reexamine what is really important to me. Everything seems more meaningful. My wife and children have always been the light of my life, but before Patty and I struggled with illness, we did not have the depth of caring and togetherness that we now share. My family, my dog, my friends, my work all seem more important to me. Since my struggles, I enjoy my grandchild with more delight than would have been possible before.

Being a patient has made me a better physician. It has broadened my professional understanding of chronic illness and our reactions to it. Watching my wife suffer with fibromyalgia changed my approach to the treatment of people with chronic pain. My own illnesses gave me more empathy. Most health care professionals change when they experience illness from the other side. Students at Harvard Medical School take a course during which they spend time as "patients," including a night in the hospital. This role-playing is a crucial first step in learning the art of the physician-patient relationship.

My illness has made me less self-absorbed and less worried about what others might think. It feels much easier to try new things since I don't care so much about being "the best." I no longer play competitive tennis and squash but enjoy such activities as a yoga class or water aerobics. Patty and I are taking ballroom dance lessons and learning golf, two activities that did not interest me before. Adapting to health uncertainty teaches flexibility.

9) Be patient since time is the great healer.

When we become ill, time seems to be our enemy. We rush around to find the right doctor and get the best treatment. During my illnesses, I kept thinking of a line from a poem by T.S. Eliot: "Hurry up please, it's time." But what is it time for?

I felt great pressure and urgency but finally realized that in chronic, non-life threatening illness, time is our ally. We are not racing a disease that could get steadily worse and even shorten our life. We do indeed have time to get better. If we stop rushing around looking for causes and blame, we'll be better off. If we stop forcing ourselves to get healthy, our natural healing powers will come into their own. Given time, they will usually bring us around.

The most precious gift of time is the opportunity to see our illness more objectively. When I made use of this opportunity by accepting my illness and "moving on" in my life, I was on the path to recovery. Full recovery will take more time and may not even be practical, but I can now accept that. I am now much more tolerant of the ups and downs in my health. Andrew Weil describes sickness as a step toward health (95). The two states are relative: one cannot exist without the other. Certainly health cannot be appreciated without having experienced illness. For a few years, my health felt like a roller coaster that kept plunging to the bottom. Now I see the "ups" as well as the "downs."

Counseling, time, and patience helped me to understand how I was reacting negatively to illness and uncertainty. People always need a period of adjustment to respond optimally to illness—or to any challenge in life. After a number of months, I began to feel better. I became convinced that I was not going to die after all! I was slowly able to reduce the large number of medications that I had been taking. Rather than obsessing about not feeling better totally and immediately—about facing one medical calamity after another—I gave myself a respite. I stopped catastrophizing. Suddenly I could see that there were other things in life beside my current medical problems and worries.

Most people with fibromyalgia and CFS do get better over time. In chronic illnesses, there is always a tremendous ebb and flow. For example, depression often comes with the stress of illness, and anti-depressant medication can help during the worse episodes. But taking such drugs for awhile does not mean you will need to take them for the rest of your life.

Think of your illness as an ocean. If you stop struggling and find peace in your condition, you will be carried along more naturally. You will ride the swells up and down, sometimes swimming and sometimes resting. You will have periods of calm when you can float along without much thought or care. You can strive for your goals or simply enjoy the beauty and the vastness and the sky overhead. But however you set your course, be prepared for the storms ahead. Whether big or small, they can come without warning or reason. Finally they will pass, leaving you more aware of the calm and beauty when it returns.

10) Life can be happy and fulfilling despite your illness.

Some patients who come to me with fibromyalgia and chronic fatigue leave my office disappointed. Some say when they first arrive, "You are my last resort." But I cannot cure fibromyalgia and its associated illnesses. I cannot even cure my own illnesses. When I explain that I do not have all the answers, patients are sometimes angry and often frustrated. They want a cure. They want to get "fixed" and be like they used to be.

What we all need to learn is how to feel better in the context of our illness, despite its new problems and fears. I hope that I can provide patients with some guidelines. But doctors can rarely "cure." Cure may not be a realistic goal in most chronic illnesses. Instead of cures, my patients and I are looking for ways they (and I) can live the most rewarding life open to us. Remember the warning of Lewis Thomas, *"We do not seem to be seeking more exuberance in living as much as staving off failure, putting off dying"* (109).

My illness has made me more resilient and even more exuberant. It has renewed a spark in me that had been lost as I pursued my profession, my intense exercise, and all my other goals. Now I appreciate life much more. I am no longer the person I was before, and I miss some things I can no longer do. But looking ahead, I feel much more confident about facing adversity. Life seems more like an adventure.

I hope that my patients will gain some of these same feelings. We cannot know the future or completely control what will happen to us. The challenge is to make the best of what comes—to live each day to our fullest. We only waste our energy and increase stress by always "waiting for the other shoe to drop."

The challenge of living with our illness may seem impossible at times, but each time we meet it, we gain strength. These illnesses may be poorly understood, but we can deal with them if we understand ourselves, our role, and our power to change.

Table 1: Classification of illness based on a scientific understanding of the pathophysiology of the illness

<u>Illnesses in which the exact cause is known:</u>
Examples: Pneumonia, bronchitis, tuberculosis, AIDS

<u>Illnesses which are partially understood, as far as pathology and physiology, but the exact cause is not known:</u>
Examples: Cancer, heart disease, hypertension, rheumatoid arthritis

<u>Illnesses that are not understood (syndromes):</u>
Examples: Fibromyalgia, chronic fatigue syndrome, migraine, chronic low back pain, irritable bowel syndrome, depression

Table 2: Ten most common, reported medical conditions*

Condition	% of Population with Condition
Back pain	20
Allergies	16
Joint and muscle pain	16
Insomnia	14
Sprains or strains	13
Headache	13
High blood pressure	11
Digestive problems	10
Anxiety	10
Depression	8

* Modified from Eisenberg, et al: *The New England Journal of Medicine,* 1993:328,246-52 (3)

Table 3: Diagnostic features of fibromyalgia, chronic fatigue syndrome (CFS), migraine, and irritable bowel syndrome (IBS)

Condition	Essential diagnostic features	Frequent other features
Fibromyalgia	Diffuse muscle pain; Multiple tender points	Fatigue, sleep disturbance Headache, IBS, Mood disturbances
CFS	Debilitating fatigue	Muscle, joint pain, Headache, difficulty concentrating, mood and sleep disturbances
Migraine	Episodic, vascular headache	Visual aura, fatigue
IBS	Abdominal pain; Diarrhea, constipation, cramps	Fatigue, sleep and mood disturbances

Table 4: Diagnostic Criteria for Major Depression

At least 5 of the following are present during the same period and symptoms are present for most of the day, nearly daily for at least 2 weeks.

Depressed mood*
Markedly diminished interest or pleasure in all
    or nearly all activities*
Significant weight loss or gain or change in
    appetite
Insomnia or hypersomnia
Psychomotor agitation or retardation
Fatigue
Feelings of worthlessness or excessive
    inappropriate guilt
Impaired concentration or indecisiveness
Recurrent thoughts of death or suicide

* Must be present for the diagnosis of depression

Table 5: Psychiatric Studies in Fibromyalgia, Chronic Fatigue Syndrome

- Most patients do not have a current psychiatric illness: 25-35% have major depression
- Many patients have modest depression and anxiety, typical of any chronic illness
- There may be a biologic predisposition to mood disturbances based on family, hormonal studies
- Pain and fatigue do not correlate well with psychologic symptoms
- "Stress" may be an important factor in expression of these illnesses

Table 6: Similar Features of Fibromyalgia and Chronic Fatigue Syndrome

- 80-90% are women; usual age of onset is 20-55 yrs
- Myalgias and fatigue are present in 90% of patients
- Associated common symptoms include neurocognitive problems, mood disturbances, headaches, sleep disturbance
- No identifiable "cause"
- Normal laboratory, radiologic tests; multiple "tender points" found on examination in all patients with fibromyalgia and the majority with chronic fatigue syndrome
- Chronic symptoms, no highly effective treatment

Table 7: Therapeutic Principles of Fibromyalgia and Chronic Fatigue Syndrome

Education
- Explain what these illnesses are and what is the typical course of these chronic disorders
- Review the importance of the mind-body interaction
- Emphasize patient's role in reaction to chronic illness

Medication
- Treat sleep disturbance
- Analgesic medications
- Consider serotonin reuptake inhibitors in selected patients

Activity-exercise program
- Appropriate rest-activity cycle
- Gentle cardiovascular fitness training
- "Hands on" physical therapy, massage, etc.

Longitudinal support
- Counseling for patient and family
- Relaxation techniques, cognitive behavior therapy

Table 8: Analgesics, anti-inflammatory medications, antidepressants and others medications useful in the treatment of chronic pain

Analgesic medications
Acetaminophen
Narcotic analgesics (e.g., Percocet, codeine)

Antiinflammatory medications
Aspirin
Non-steroidal antiinflammatory medications
(e.g., ibuprofen, naproxen, indomethacin)
Corticosteroids (used orally, e.g., prednisone, or by injection)

Antidepressants
Tricyclic antidepressants (e.g. Elavil)
Serotonin-reuptake inhibitors (e.g. Prozac, Zoloft, Paxil)

Others
Medicines more often used to treat anxiety:
(e.g.. Xanax, Klonopin, Ativan, Valium)
"Muscle relaxants": (e.g., Flexeril, Soma, Robaxin)
Neuroleptics (e.g., Dilantin, Depakote, Tegretol)
Selective medications: (e.g., sumatriptan and ergot alkaloids for the treatment of migraine; beta blockers and other medications for the prevention of migraine).

Table 9: Medications for the treatment of mood and sleep disturbances

Medications	*Comments*
Treatment of depression	
Tricyclics, including amitriptyline (Elavil), nortriptyline (Pamelor), imipramine (Tofranil)	Effective but frequent dry mouth, grogginess; low doses useful for sleep disturbances
Trazodone (Desyrel)	Mechanism of action not clear; less side effects than tricyclics; useful for sleep disturbances
Nefazodone (Serzone)	Similar, but less side effects than trazodone; new drug on market
Selective serotonin reuptake inhibitors, including fluoxetine (Prozac), sertraline (Zoloft), paroxetine (Paxil), fluvoxamine (Luvox)	Excellent antidepressants with less side effects than tricyclics or MAO inhibitors
Monoamine oxidase (MAO) inhibitors (Nardil)	Used only when failure of SSRI's or tricyclics, because of greater side effects and more interactions with food, etc.
Venlafaxine (Effexor)	Inhibits both serotonin and norepinephrine uptake
Bupropion (Wellbutrin)	Inhibits norepinephrine. Usually well-tolerated

Treatment of anxiety

Antidepressants	Many of the above are also helpful for treatment of anxiety
Benzodiazepines, such as clonazepam (Klonopin), lorazepam (Ativan), alprazolam (Xanax)	Difficult to withdraw from these agents; very useful for insomnia

Treatment of insomnia

Antidepressants and anti-anxiety agents may be helpful	Often best choice because of common association of mood and sleep disturbances
Hypnotics, including triazolam (Halcion), temazepam (Restoril) flurazepam (Dalmane)	All benzodiazepines and similar sleeping pills may be habit-forming
Zolpidem (Ambien)	Non-benzodiazepines hypnotic. Less habit-forming.

Table 10. Alternative medicine used by 80 patients with fibromyalgia*

Therapy	% using	Satisfaction†
Over-the counter items	70	5
Creams, rubs	50	
Vitamins	35	
Herbal products	29	
Spiritual practices	48	9
Prayers	41	
Meditation	38	
Relaxation	10	
Self-help group	6	
Spiritual healing	5	
Practitioners	40	8
Chiropractor	19	
Massage	10	
Acupuncture	8	
Homeopathy	4	
Reflexology	3	
Dietary modifications	26	5
Additions to diet	20	
Subtractions from diet	25	

* Modified from Pioro-Boisset, et al: Alternative Medicine Use in Fibromyalgia Syndrome. *Arthritis Care and Research* 1996;9:15
† Average score from 0 to 10, with 10=most satisfied

Figure 1: A Psychosocial Model of Fibromyalgia*

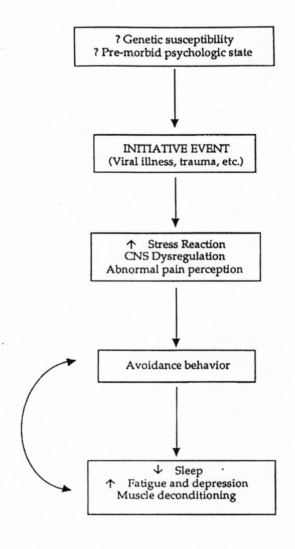

*Modified from: Goldenberg, D. What is the future of fibromyalgia? Rheum Dis Clin N Amer 22; 1996, 395.

Figure 2: Location of tender points in fibromyalgia*

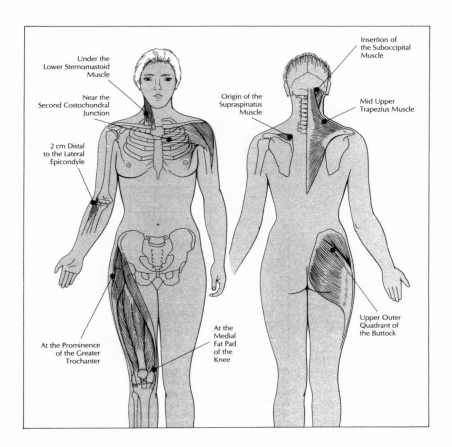

*From: Goldenberg, D. Diagnostic and Therapeutic Challenges of Fibro-myalgia. Hospital Practice 24; 1989, 45.

Figure 3: Common syndromes that overlap with fibromyalgia.*

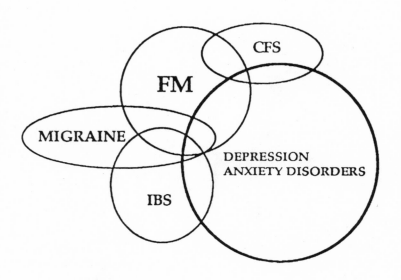

FM = Fibromyalgia
CFS = chronic fatigue syndrome
IBS = irritable bowel syndrome

*Modified from: Goldenberg, D. What is the future of fibromyalgia? Rheum Dis Clin N Amer 22; 1996, 397.

REFERENCES AND NOTES

1. Jiang W. Babyak M, Krantz DS, et al: Mental stress-induced myocardial ischemia and cardiac events. JAMA 275:1651,-56, 1996
This research demonstrated that mental, as well as physical stress, reduces blood flow to the heart. Mental stress was also associated with an increased risk for a heart attack. Therefore, we should attempt to modify the stress levels of people with cardiac disease. Stress-reduction techniques may be as important as cardiovascular fitness training in the prevention of heart attacks.

2. Muller JE, Mittleman MA, Maclure M, Sherwood JB, Tofler GH: Triggering myocardial infarction by sexual activity. JAMA 275:1405-9, 1996
In this study, 1774 patients who had just experienced a heart attack were interviewed and asked about potential triggers of their heart attacks. There was a very low risk of triggering a heart attack by sexual activity. The absolute risk was about one in a million and that risk was not increased in patients with a prior history of cardiac disease. Regular exercise programs decreased the risk of sexual activity triggering heart attacks.

3. Eisenberg DM, Kessler RC, Foster C, Norlock FE, Calkins DR, Delbanco TL: Unconventional medicine in the United States. Prevalence, costs, and patterns in use. N Eng J Med 328:246-252, 1993
Eisenberg and colleagues surveyed a random sample of the population at large to determine their use of unconventional

or non-traditional care for the most common health problems. The 10 most common medical disorders (depicted in Table 2) are poorly understood and primarily represent syndromes, rather than diseases. They include most of the illnesses discussed in this book. One-third of the Americans surveyed had used non-traditional therapy for the treatment of these common syndromes, such as back pain, headaches and insomnia. A vast amount of American dollars is spent for non-traditional treatment of our health despite little evidence that this treatment is very effective.

4. Yunus M, Masi AT, Calabro JJ, Miller KA, Feigenbaum SL: Primary fibromyalgia (fibrositis): clinical study of 50 patients with matched normal controls. Semin Arthritis Rheum 11:151-171, 1981
Yunus compared 50 patients with fibromyalgia with 50 age and sex matched controls. He focused on the clinical features that were helpful in the diagnosis of fibromyalgia. This was one of the first modern studies that got rheumatologists interested in fibromyalgia.

5. Goldenberg DL: What is the future of fibromyalgia? Rheum Dis Clin N Amer 22:393-406, 1996
I discuss a number of different current avenues of research in fibromyalgia. There are a number of precipitating events that seem to trigger fibromyalgia. The future of fibromyalgia research will focus on the central nervous system. More longitudinal studies need to be done and subsets of patients should be evaluated. Rheumatologists will be used more as consultants than primary care physicians in the treatment of fibromyalgia.

6. Wolfe F, Smythe HA, Yunus MB, Bennett RM, Bombardier C, Goldenberg DL, Tugwell P, Campbell SM, Abeles M, Clark P, Fam AG, Farber SJ, Fiechtner JJ, Franklin CM, Gatter RA, Hamaty D, Lessard J, Lichtbroun AS, Masi AT, McCain GA, Reynolds WJ, Romano TJ, Russell IJ, Sheon RP: The

American College of Rheumatology 1990 criteria for the classification of fibromyalgia: Report of the Multicenter Criteria Committee. Arthritis Rheum 33:160-172, 1990
This multi-center study compared a large group of patients felt to have fibromyalgia with other patients with chronic painful rheumatic disorders. History, physical examination and laboratory findings were compared in the two groups to obtain classification criteria for the diagnosis of fibromyalgia. Those diagnostic criteria that provided the best sensitivity and specificity for the classification of fibromyalgia were chronic, diffuse pain and at least 11 of 18 pre-defined tender points. These criteria have been very useful in clinical trials and epidemiologic studies. However, they are not as useful in certain settings and patients may have fibromyalgia and not meet this definition.

7. Goldenberg DL: Fibromyalgia syndrome. An emerging but controversial condition. JAMA 257:2782-2787, 1987
This was the first review article on fibromyalgia that appeared in a widely read general medical journal. It discussed the major clinical manifestations of fibromyalgia and explored the controversial nature of the disorder.

8. Dinerman H, Goldenberg DL, Felson DT: A prospective evaluation of 118 patients with the fibromyalgia syndrome: prevalence of Raynaud's phenomenon, sicca symptoms, ANA, low complement, and Ig deposition at the dermal-epidermal junction. J Rheumatol 13:368-373, 1986
Symptoms that are often found in immunologic and connective tissue diseases may also be found in fibromyalgia. These include the symptoms of Raynaud's phenomenon and dryness of the eyes and mouth. However, rarely do patients with typical fibromyalgia later develop one of the immunologic or connective tissue diseases, provided there was initially no clinical evidence of such disorders. Some patients will also have positive blood tests, such as a positive antinuclear antibody test, although these positive tests occur no more often in fibromyalgia than in the normal population.

9. Simms RW, Goldenberg DL: Symptoms mimicking neurologic disorders in fibromyalgia syndrome. J. Rheumatol 15:1271-1273, 1988
Numbness and tingling of the extremities is common in fibromyalgia. These symptoms suggest the possibility of a neurologic disorders, such as carpal tunnel syndrome or a cervical radiculopathy. However, generally the neurologic symptoms do not reflect nerve damage or pathology. However, fibromyalgia patients often undergo needless testing and sometimes unnecessary surgery because of the failure to suspect fibromyalgia as the cause of these symptoms.

10. Marder WD, Meenan RF, Felson DT, Reichlin M, Birnbaum NS, Croft JD, Dore RK, Kaplan H, Kaufman RL, Stobo JD: Editorial: The present and future adequacy of rheumatology manpower: A study of health care needs and physician supply. Arthritis Rheum 34:1209-1217, 1991
After osteoarthritis, fibromyalgia is the most common rheumatic disorder. For physicians, fibromyalgia takes up the second most time in rheumatology practice, exceeded only by rheumatoid arthritis.

11. Goldenberg DL: Fibromyalgia: why such controversy? Ann Rheum Dis 54:3-5, 1995
This editorial discusses the persistent controversy about the existence of fibromyalgia as a discrete syndrome. There is evidence that the diagnostic label does more good for people suffering from this disorder than proposed harm.

12. Buchwald D: Fibromyalgia and chronic fatigue syndrome. Rheum Dis Clin N Amer 22:219-243, 1996
The clinical similarities of fibromyalgia and CFS are compared and contrasted. There are striking similar demographic, clinical and laboratory feature of these two conditions.

13. Hudson JI, Hudson MS, Pliner LF, Goldenberg DL, Pope HG,Jr.: Fibromyalgia and major affective disorder: a controlled phenomenology and family history study. AM J Psychiatry 142:441-446, 1985

A group of patients with fibromyalgia and with rheumatoid arthritis received a structured psychiatric interview which generated a diagnosis of current and past psychiatric illness. There was a greater personal and family history of depression in fibromyalgia compared to rheumatoid arthritis patients. However, only 30% of patients were depressed at the time of the diagnosis of fibromyalgia.

14. Goldenberg DL: An overview of psychologic studies in fibromyalgia. J Rheumatol 16 Suppl. 19:12-14, 1989
This article reviews the studies that have evaluated psychologic symptoms and psychiatric illness in patients with fibromyalgia. There is greater personal stress and hassles in people with fibromyalgia than in the normal population. The majority of research studies suggest that there is a biologic link of mood disturbances with fibromyalgia. However, only 20-35% of fibromyalgia patients have current major depression.

15. Hudson JI, Goldenberg DL, Pope HG,Jr., Keck PE,Jr., Schlesinger L: Comorbidity of fibromyalgia with medical and psychiatric disorders. Am J Med 92:363-367, 1992
Structured interviews of patients with fibromyalgia found that there was a significant overlap with the other syndromes discussed in this book. Fibromyalgia commonly is associated with chronic fatigue syndrome, migraine, irritable bowel syndrome and depression. It is not clear whether this overlap represents common external factors or a biologic predisposition.

16. Goldenberg DL, Felson DT, Dinerman H: A randomized, controlled trial of amitriptyline and naproxen in the treatment of patients with fibromyalgia. Arthritis Rheum 29:1371-1377, 1986
This study found that low doses of amitriptyline (25 mgs at bedtime) were modestly effective in patients with fibromyalgia. However, the anti-inflammatory medication naprosyn (500 mgs twice daily) was no better in the treatment of fibromyalgia than a placebo. A combination of the two medications was better for pain relief than the amitriptyline alone.

17. Goldenberg DL, Mayskiy M, Mossey CJ, Ruthazer R, Schmid C: A randomized, double-blind crossover trial of fluoxetine and amitriptyline in the treatment of fibromyalgia. Arthritis Rheum 39:1852-1859, 1996
We compared the efficacy of 20 mgs of fluoxetine (Prozac) to 25 mgs of amitriptyline (Elavil) in the treatment of fibromyalgia. The two drugs equally improved the pain and overall well being in fibromyalgia. Both worked better than a placebo. The combination of the two worked better than either alone. This may relate to the different chemical effects that such medications have on the central nervous system, especially on increasing the bioavailability of serotonin.

18. Buchwald D, Goldenberg DL, Sullivan JL, Komaroff AL: The "chronic, active Epstein-Barr virus infection: syndrome and primary fibromyalgia. Arthritis Rheum 30:1132-1136, 1987
This was the initial report that described the overlap of symptoms of fibromyalgia with those of chronic fatigue syndrome. The results led to our hypothesis that these two syndromes may represent manifestation of the same illness.

19. Goldenberg DL, Simms RW, Geiger A, Komaroff AL: High frequency of fibromyalgia in patients with chronic fatigue seen in a primary care practice. Arthritis Rheum 33:381-387, 1990
We examined a group of patients who had been followed in a chronic fatigue syndrome clinic to determine how many of them had symptoms and signs of fibromyalgia. Seventy percent of patients with chronic fatigue syndrome had tender points and met the diagnostic criteria for fibromyalgia.

20. Triadafilopoulos G, Simms RW, Goldenberg DL: Bowel dysfunction in fibromyalgia syndrome. Dig Dis Sci 36:59-64, 1991
Approximately 70% of patients with fibromyalgia meet the clinical criteria for the diagnosis of irritable bowel syndrome. Similar demographic and clinical profiles are found in each of these disorders.

21. Russell IJ, Orr MD, Littman B, Vipraio GA, Alboufrek D, Michalek JE, Lopez Y, MacKillip F: Elevated cerebrospinal fluid levels of substance P in patients with the fibromyalgia syndrome. Arthritis Rheum 37:1593-1601, 1994
The level of substance P was higher in the spinal fluid of fibromyalgia patients than in normal controls. Substance P is an important determinant of pain sensitivity.

22. Bennett RM, Clark SR, Campbell SM, Burckhardt CS: Low levels of somatomedin-C in patients with the fibromyalgia syndrome: a possible link between sleep and muscle pain. Arthritis Rheum 35:1113-1116, 1992
Low levels of somatomedin C, which reflects levels of growth hormone, were found in some patients with fibromyalgia. Growth hormone is important in the function of homeostasis of muscle. Growth hormone is secreted primarily during deep sleep and is affected by sleep disturbances. Although this is a very important finding, growth hormone testing can not be used to diagnosis fibromyalgia.

23. Griep EN, Boersma JW, de Kloet ER: Altered reactivity of the hypothalmic-pituitary-adrenal axis in the primary fibromyalgia syndrome. J Rheumatol 20:469-474, 1993
Abnormal hypothalamic-pituitary-adrenal axis hormones status was found in some fibromyalgia patients. These are the cortisol and "fight or flight" related compounds.

24. Simms RW, Roy SH, Hrovat M, Anderson JJ, Skrinar G, LePoole SR, Zerbini CAF, De Luca C, Jolesz F: Lack of association between fibromyalgia syndrome and abnormalities in muscle energy metabolism. Arthritis Rheum 37:794-800, 1994
This study compared muscle function and metabolism during exercise in fibromyalgia patients and sedentary controls. MRI spectroscopy was used in a very sophisticated analysis. No evidence for muscle hypoxia or abnormal muscle metabolism was found. Similar findings by other groups leads to the conclusion that the pain and weakness felt in fibromyalgia muscle is not related to direct muscle damage or pathology.

25. Russell IJ, Vaeroy H, Javors M, Nyberg F: Cerebrospinal fluid biogenic amine metabolites in fibromyalgia/fibrositis syndrome and rheumatoid arthritis. Arthritis Rheum 35:550-556, 1992
Certain proteins and amino acids were found to be of different concentrations in the cerebrospinal fluid of patients with fibromyalgia compared to rheumatoid arthritis controls. Such substances may be important in pain, sleep and energy.

26. Goldenberg DL: A review of the role of tricyclic medications in the treatment of fibromyalgia syndrome. J Rheumatol Suppl 19:137-139, 1989
Tricyclic medications, such as amitriptyline and cyclobenzaprine, have been shown to be of modest benefit in controlled clinical trials in fibromyalgia. These medications are used in low dose and generally taken before bedtime. They usually are well tolerated but can cause constipation, weight gain and lethargy. The mechanism of action of these medicines in fibromyalgia is not understood although they affect pain perception and sleep.

27. McCain GA: A cost-effective approach to the diagnosis and treatment of fibromyalgia. Rheum Dis Clin N Amer 22:323-349, 1996
This review presents a practical guideline for the evaluation and treatment of patients with fibromyalgia. Cost-effectiveness is best maintained if the physician thinks of the diagnosis early.

28. Bennett RM, Campbell S, Burckhardt C, Clark SR, O'Reilly C, Weins A: A multidisciplinary approach to fibromyalgia treatment. J Musculoskel Med 8:21-32, 1991
A multidisciplinary team approach was quite effective in the treatment of fibromyalgia. Education, physical therapy, counseling and medications are used together in such an approach.

29. Kaplan KH, Goldenberg DL, Galvin-Nadeau M: The impact of a meditation-based stress reduction program on fibromyalgia. Gen Hosp Psychiat 15:284-289, 1993

A meditation-based relaxation response program was found to help reduce the symptoms of fibromyalgia. Patients were taught relaxation techniques such as meditation and yoga and were also taught how to best cope with the illness by modifying their behavior. Such programs have also been useful in the treatment of chronic fatigue syndrome, migraine and insomnia.

30. Granges G, Zilko P, Littlejohn GO: Fibromyalgia syndrome: assessment of the severity of the condition 2 years after diagnosis. J Rheumatol 21:523-529, 1994
This is the only study to date that measured the outcome of patients with fibromyalgia treated by generalists and not by specialists. The outcome in general was quite good with one-quarter of patients having a complete remission and most patients doing well with minimal intervention.

31. Pawlikowska T, Chalder T, Hirsch SR, Wallace P, Wright DJM, Wessely SC: Population based study of fatigue and psychological distress. BMJ 308:763-766, 1994
Most population based studies have found a 10-20% prevalence of chronic fatigue, as did this report. There was a strong correlation of fatigue with psychological distress. Most people with chronic fatigue do not meet the definition criteria of CFS.

32. Goldenberg DL: Fatigue in rheumatic disease. Bull Rheum Dis 44:4-8, 1995
The definition of fatigue and ways to measure its severity are discussed. Fatigue is an important symptom in the classic immune disorders such as lupus and rheumatoid arthritis. It is also one of the characteristic symptoms of fibromyalgia, CFS and depression.

33. Beard GM: Neurasthenia, or nervous exhaustion. Boston Medical and Surgical Journal 3:217-221, 1869
George Beard was the first physician to popularize the illness termed neurasthenia. His accounts of the symptoms of that condition are very similar to symptoms of chronic fatigue and fibromyalgia syndromes.

34. Goldenberg DL: Fibromyalgia and other chronic fatigue syndromes: is there evidence for chronic viral illness? Semin Arthritis Rheum 18:111-120, 1988
This review traces the historical similarity of fibromyalgia and chronic fatigue syndrome. Epidemics of chronic fatigue syndrome which may have been triggered by an infectious agent are discussed.

35. Komaroff AL, Goldenberg D: The chronic fatigue syndrome: definition, current studies and lessons for fibromyalgia research. J Rheumatol Suppl 19:23-27, 1989
Clinical and laboratory features of fibromyalgia overlap considerably.

36. Goldenberg DL: Fibromyalgia and its relation to chronic fatigue syndrome, viral illness and immune abnormalities. J Rheumatol 16 (Suppl. 19):91-93, 1989
This review discuss the epidemics of chronic fatigue and the possible relationship of these epidemics with infections.The symptoms described by patients during these epidemics and the clinical course that their illness followed are similar to fibromyalgia and chronic fatigue syndrome.

37. Acheson ED: The clinical syndrome variously called benign myalgic encephalomyelitis, Iceland disease, and epidemic neuromyasthenia. Am J Med 26:569-595, 1959
This extensive review traces outbreaks of BME, now known as CFS. Most of these epidemic occurred in the 1930s. In reading the symptoms and clinical course of the 1000 patients in these epidemics, there are striking similarities to the Lake Tahoe and other epidemics of CFS described in the 1980s.

38. Scott S, Deary I, Pelosi AJ: General practitioners' attitudes to patients with a self diagnosis of myalgic encephalomyelitis. BMJ 310:861-864, 1995
The term BME is still used in the United Kingdom. Most practitioners are not using that diagnosis. Many support groups however still are called BME patient support groups. Many

general physicians do not use that diagnosis and are not convinced that the condition is real.

39. Straus SE, Tosato G, Armstrong G, Lawley T, Preble OT, Henle W, Davey R, Pearson G, Epstein J, Brus I, Blaese M: Persisting illness and fatigue in adults with evidence of Epstein-Barr virus infection. Ann Intern Med 102:7-16, 1985
Two groups reported clusters of cases in the United States of patients with chronic fatigue, myalgias and neurocognitive symptoms. The average antibody levels to antigens found on the Epstein-Barr virus were greater in these patients than in matched controls. This was the most influential study that suggested that CFS was a discrete illness and might be caused by a virus.

40. Buchwald D, Cheney PR, Peterson DL, Henry B, Wormsley SB, Geiger A, Ablashi DV, Salahuddin Z, Saxinger C, Biddle R, Kikinis R, Jolesz FA, Folks T, Balachandran N, Peter JB, Gallo RC, Konaroff AL: A chronic illness characterized by fatigue, neurologic and immunologic disorders, and active human herpesvirus type 6 infection. Ann Intern Med 116:103-113, 1992
Extensive research proved that the Epstein-Barr virus was not the cause of most cases of CFS. Other viruses have been incriminated, including a group of herpesviruses, although most investigators believe that no single infectious agent will be directly involved in most cases of CFS.

41. Holmes GP, Kaplan JE, Gantz NM, Komaroff AL, Schonberger LB, Straus SE, Jones JF, Dubois RE, Cunningham-Rundles C, Pahwa S, Tosato G, Zegans LS, Purtilo DT, Brown N, Schooley RT, Brus I: Chronic fatigue syndrome: a working case definition. Ann Intern Med 108:387-389, 1988
This was the first case definition of chronic fatigue syndrome, although it was subsequently revised to be less restrictive. The definition included the debilitating fatigue but insisted on a group of other symptoms and on excluding illnesses such as depression.

42. Schluederberg A, Straus SE, Peterson P, Blumenthal S, Komaroff AL, Spring SB, Landay A, Buchwald D: Chronic fatigue syndrome research. Definition and medical outcome assessment. Ann Intern Med 117:325-331, 1992
This reports further described the evolution of the working case definition for CFS. A group of experts met and determined which symptoms and findings were most helpful in differentiating CFS from other causes of chronic fatigue. These definitions have been modified and are broader than when first proposed. Fibromyalgia, depression and anxiety are not exclusions to the diagnosis of CFS.

43. Dinerman H, Steere AC: Lyme disease associated with fibromyalgia. Ann Intern Med 117:281-285, 1992
Fibromyalgia was found to be common after Lyme disease was treated. The infection that causes Lyme disease may be a precipitating factor in fibromyalgia and CFS.

44. Steere AC, Taylor E, McHugh GL, Logigian EL: The overdiagnosis of Lyme disease. JAMA 269:1812-1816, 1993
Steere found that only 25% of patients referred to his clinic had Lyme disease. Many of these people who were misdiagnosed or thought that they had Lyme disease had chronic fatigue syndrome/fibromyalgia. He also demonstrated that CFS, as well as fibromyalgia, frequently follow well-documented Lyme disease. These chronic symptoms do not respond to antibiotics and are not felt to be related to persistent Lyme infection.

45. Schwartz RB, Komaroff AL, Garada BM, Gleit M, Doolittle TH, Bates DW, Vasile RG, Holman BL: SPECT imaging of the brain: Comparison of findings in patients with chronic fatigue syndrome, AIDS dementia complex, and major unipolar depression. Am J Radiol 162:943-951, 1994
Blood flow abnormalities to the brain were found in some patients with CFS. These changes were different than the findings in patients with depression and AIDS.

46. Demitrack MA, Dale JK, Straus SE, Laue L, Listwak SJ, Kruesi MJP, Chrousos GP, Gold PW: Evidence for impaired

activation of the hypothalamic-pituitary-adrenal axis in patients with chronic fatigue syndrome. J Clin Endocrinol Metab 73:1224-1234, 1991
An expertly done study that demonstrated subtle endocrine abnormalities in some patients with CFS. The changes primarily were in the hypothalamic-pituatary-adrenal axis.

47. Bou-Holaigah I, Rowe PC, Kan J, Calkins H: The relationship between neurally mediated hypotension and the chronic fatigue syndrome. JAMA 274:961-967, 1995
Upright tilt table testing for the presence of neurally mediated hypotension was performed in 23 patients with CFS and 14 healthy control subjects. An abnormal response was much more common in the CFS patients. This suggests that the chronic fatigue may be related to hypotension. Treatment with increased dietary salt or fludrocortisone improved symptoms in nine of nineteen patients.

48. Johnson H: Osler's Web. New York, Crown, 1996
This is a fascinating and detailed recounting of the modern-day history of chronic fatigue syndrome. However, it provides a biased focus on the scientific communities' lack of compassion and at time blind refusal to accept CFS as a infectious disease that "can devastate the immune system and attack the brain."

49. Bombardier CH, Buchwald D: Outcome and prognosis of patients with chronic fatigue vs. chronic fatigue syndrome. Arch Intern Med 155:2105-10, 1995
Four-hundred and ninety-eight patients with chronic fatigue or CFS who were referred to a specialist were re-evaluated at an average of 1.5 years. Sixty-four percent reported improvement but only 2% reported complete resolution of all CFS symptoms. At follow-up, CFS patients reported more symptoms and greater disability than patients with chronic fatigue who did not meet CFS criteria. Depression predicted poor outcome.

50. Deyo RA, Diehl AK: Psychosocial predictors of disability in patients with low back pain. J Rheumatol 15:1557-1564, 1988

Psychosocial factors, such as the workplace setting and level of education, are the most important predictors of disability in people with low back pain. The importance of these factors has also been demonstrated in rheumatoid arthritis and fibromyalgia.

51. von Korff M, Deyo RA, Cherkin D, Barlow W: Back pain in primary care. Outcomes at 1 year. Spine 18:855-862, 1993

This report looks at the outcome of back pain when seen by primary care physicians. Ninety percent of patients with acute back pain seen in this setting have complete resolution of their pain within one year. Generally back pain subsides on its own without any major treatment. Nevertheless, the 10% of people who continue to have back pain represent a very large number of patients in the United States.

52. Jensen MC, Brant-Zawadzki MN, Obuchowski N, Modic MT, Malkasian D, Ross JS: Magnetic resonance imaging of the lumbar spine in people without back pain. N Engl J Med 331:69-73, 1994

Fifty-two percent of people without any back pain had a disc bulge demonstrated by MRI. Twenty-seven percent had a disc protrusion. Thus the finding of disc bulges or protrusions in people with back pain may frequently be coincidental.

53. Kabat-Zinn J: Full Catastrophe Living. New York, Delta, 1990

Full Catastrophe Living describes the program used by Zinn in the stress reduction clinic at the University of Massachusetts Medical Center. It is an excellent resource for understanding all aspects of the practice of mindfulness. My colleagues and I have patterned our own mind-body course after Dr Zinn's. There are extended instructions in meditation, yoga and various stressors.

54. Kabat-Zinn J: Wherever You Go, There You Are. New York, Hyperion, 1994
This is a beautifully written book describing how mindfulness can lead us to happier and more peaceful lives. It flows like poetry and philosophy, chock full of useful and practical advice on expanding our view of the world and how we connect to it.

55. Hauri P, Linde S: No More Sleepless Nights. New York, John Wiley and Sons, 1990
This is an excellent, detailed book about all forms of sleep disturbances. It also contains practical guides about treatment, especially non-medicinal approaches to improved sleep.

56. Borbély A: Secrets of Sleep. Stuttgart, Basic Books, 1984
A scholarly review of sleep, with special emphasis on the neuroanatomy of normal and abnormal sleep.

57. Moldofsky H, Lue FA, Davidson JR, Gorczynski R: Effects of sleep deprivation on human immune functions. FASEB Journal 3:1972-1977, 1989
Sleep and sleep deprivation were studied. There are notable effects of sleep deprivation on mood and our immune systems.

58. Davidson JR, Moldofsky H, Lue FA: Growth hormone and coritsol secretion in relation to sleep and wakefulness. J Psychiatr Neurosci 16:96-102, 1991
Moldofsky and co-workers were the first investigators to report that most patients with fibromyalgia have abnormal deep sleep, with frequent alpha wave interruption of delta sleep.

59. Moldofsky H, Lue FA, Eisen J, Keystone E, Gorczynski RM: The relationship of interleukin-1 and immune functions to sleep in humans. Psychosom Med 48:309-318, 1986
These same investigators have studied the physiologic, chemical and immunologic changes that occur at various stages of sleep.

60. Strollo PJ, Rogers RM: Obstructive sleep apnea. N Engl J Med 334-99-104, 1996
This reviews the pathophysiology and treatment of obstructive sleep apnea. Medications have not been very helpful. First-line treatment is positive pressure via a mask worn during the night. Surgery may be required in severe cases.

61. Young T, Palta M, Dempsey J, Skatrud J, Weber S, Badr S: The occurrence of sleep-disordered breathing among middle-age adults. N Engl J Med 328:1230-1235, 1993
An epidemiologic study that documented the frequency of sleep apnea and has made physicians and the public more aware of its importance.

62. Moldofsky H: Nonrestorative sleep and symptoms after a febrile illness in patients with fibrositis and chronic fatigue syndromes. J Rheumatol Suppl 19:150-153, 1989
Moldofsky reviews the evidence for similar sleep disturbances in patients with fibromyalgia and chronic fatigue syndrome.

63. O'Keefe ST: Restless leg syndrome. Arch Intern Med 156:243-248, 1996
This paper reviews the clinical manifestations of restless leg syndrome. Sleep is disturbed by involuntary movements of the extremities, often with unpleasant spasms and burning sensations. Various medicinal treatments may be useful, including levodopa, bromocriptine, clonazepam, carbamazepine and clonidine.

64. Peled R, Lavie P: Double-blind evaluation of clonazepem on periodic leg movements in sleep. J Neurol Neurosurg Psych 50:1679-1681, 1987
This controlled study demonstrated that clonazepam, at doses of 0.5-2 mg per night, was very effective in the treatment of periodic leg movements during sleep.

65. Schenck CH, Mahowald MW: Long-term, nightly benzodiazepine treatment of injurious parasomnias and other disorders of disrupted nocturnal sleep in 170 adults. Am J Med 100:333-337, 1996

Long-term nightly doses of benzodiazepines were very effective with few adverse side affects in patients with a variety of long-standing sleep disorders. Most patients were treated with clonazepam, at a mean dose of 0.77 mg for an average of 3.5 years. Eighty-six percent of patients had complete or substantial control of the sleep disorder. Only 2% abused or misused the medication. There was no significant increase in the dose of medication used over the 3.5 years.

66. Jacobs GD, Benson H, Friedman R: Perceived benefits in a behavioral-medicine insomnia program: A clinical report. Am J Med 100:212-216, 1996
Chronic insomnia patients derived significant benefit from a behavioral medicine program. Ninety percent of the patients were able to eliminate or reduce medication use for insomnia.

67. Lynn RB, Friedman LS: Current concepts: Irritable bowel syndrome. N Eng J Med 329:1940-1945, 1993
Irritable bowel syndrome occurs in 10-22% of adults. It is one of a group of disorders termed functional because no structural or organic basis has been found. Other functional disorders that cause abdominal pain include biliary dyskinesia, esophageal spasm and nonulcer dyspepsia. Pathophysiology is felt to involve disordered bowel motility and altered visceral pain sensation. Psychosocial factors are important in health care seeking.

68. Drossman DA, Thompson WG: The irritable bowel syndrome: review and a graduated multicomponent treatment approach. Ann Intern Med 116:1009-1016, 1992
Treatment that includes a multi-disciplinary physical and psychologic approach is recommended.

69. Boisset-Pioro MH, Esdaile JM, Fitzcharles M-A: Sexual and physical abuse in women with fibromyalgia syndrome. Arthritis Rheum 38:235-241, 1995
There was a modest increase in physical and sexual abuse in women with fibromyalgia compared to controls.

70. Aaron LA, Bradley LA, Alarcon GS, Alexander RW, Triana-Alexander M, Martin MY, Alberts KR: Psychiatric diagnoses in patients with fibromyalgia are related to health care-seeking behavior rather than to illness. Arthritis Rheum 39:436-445, 1996

Patients with fibromyalgia seen in a tertiary referral clinic had a significantly greater number of psychiatric diagnoses and psychologic distress than community residents who had fibromyalgia but who had not sought medical care for their symptoms. These fibromyalgia "nonpatients" did not differ from controls in psychiatric diagnoses. These results suggest that psychiatric illness is not intrinsically related to fibromyalgia, but may contribute to health care seeking.

71. Tooney TC, Seville JL, Mann D, Abashian S, Grant JR: Relationship of sexual and physical abuse to pain description, coping, psychological distress, and health-care utilization in a chronic pain sample. Clinical J Pain 11:307-315, 1995

Patients with chronic pain and a history of physical or sexual abuse had more problems coping and more psychological stress than chronic pain patients who did not have a history of such abuse. This study underscores the association of chronic pain with a history of sexual and/or physical abuse.

72. Sacks O: Migraine. Berkeley, University of California Press, 1992

This is an updated version of Sacks' original book on migraine. It is an outstanding treatise on the subject. Sacks is the neurologist who has written about his scientific observations that have become popular reading in the general public, including "Awakenings". That book was made into a successful movie with Robin Williams playing Sacks. His latest best-seller, "An Anthropologist on Mars", describes a number of his most unusual cases.

73. Diamond S, Dalessio DJ: The Practicing Physician's Approach to Headache. 3rd edition. Baltimore, Williams and Wilkins, 1982

This is a good general review of the commonest types of headaches, including diagnosis and treatment principles.

74. Stewart WF, Lipton RB, Celentano DD, et al: Age and sex-specific incidence rates of migraine with and without visual aura. Am J Epidemiol 134:1111-1115, 1991
This epidemiologic study found that 18% of females and 6% of males in the United States were suffering from migraine.

75. Olesen J: Understanding the biologic basis of migraine. N Engl J Med 331:1713-1714, 1994
Olesen reviews the evidence that migraine is a biologic disease. Studies of regional blood flow have demonstrated decreased cerebral blood supply, especially in migraine with aura. This includes a recent study using positive-emission tomography (PET scans). Involvement of serotonin locally also affects blood vessels, likely causing constriction of cerebral arteries. There is also evidence of genetic factors.

76. Sicuteri F, Anselmi B, Del Bene E, Galli P: 5-Hydroxy-tryptamine and pain modulation in man: a clinical pharmacological approach with tryptophan and parachlorophenylalanine. Acta Vitaminol Enzymol 29:66-68, 1975
A drug that effects tryptophan metabolism induced a severe pain reaction. This reaction had similar clinical features to fibromyalgia.

77. Cady RK, Wendt JK, Kirchner JR, et al: Treatment of acute migraine with subcutaneous sumatriptan. JAMA 265:2831-2836, 1991
Sumatriptan, brand name Imitrex, is a highly selective serotonin agonist which has been shown to abort attacks of migraine. It may work via selective constriction of blood flow. The medication is now available in pill or injectable form.

78. Potter WZ, Manji HK, Rudorder MV: Tricyclics and tetracyclics, Textbook of Psychopharmacology. Edited by AF Schatzberg, CB Nemeroff. Washington, DC, American Psychiatric Press, 1995 p. 141

Tricyclic medications, such as amitriptyline, have analgesic, as well as antidepressant effects. This book provides the reader with an extensive reference manual of the use and toxicity of these medications.

79. Radanov BP, Dvorak J, Valach L: Cognitive deficits in patients after soft-tissue injury of the cervical spine. Spine 17:127-31, 1992
After a muscular injury to the head and neck, many people develop problems with their memory and with intellect. The cause of these symptoms is uncertain.

80. Costa DC, Tannock C, Brostoff J: Brainstem perfusion is impaired in chronic fatigue syndrome. Quarterly J Med 88:767-73, 1995
Blood flow to the brain was decreased in patients with CFS. These are dynamic changes that may fluctuate and correct themselves.

81. Mountz JM, Bradley LA, Modell JG, Alexander RW, Triana-Alexander M, Aaron LA, Stewart KE, Alarcon GS, Mountz JD: Fibromyalgia in women. Abnormalities of regional cerebral blood flow in the thalamus and the caudate nucleus are associated with low pain threshold levels. Arthritis Rheum 38:926-938, 1995
Decreased blood flow to portions of the brain that influence pain perception, the thalami and caudate nucleus, were found in patients with fibromyalgia. This is the initial study to demonstrate a structural change in the central nervous system that may correlate with chronic pain in fibromyalgia.

82. Davies RA, Luxon LM: Dizziness following head injury: a neuro-otological study. J Neurol 242:222-30, 1996
Fifty patients with post-traumatic dizziness and a medico-legal claim were compared to 50 patients with post-traumatic dizziness not presenting for medico-legal purposes. Ninety percent of both groups had at least one audio-vestibular test abnormality. The most common was benign positional

paroxysmal vertigo. There was no difference in those patients who were seeking a medical-legal claim from the others.

83. Ash-Bernal R, Wall C,3rd, Komaroff AL, Bell D, Oas JG, Payman RN, Fagioli LR: Vestibular function test anomalies in patients with chronic fatigue syndrome. Acta Oto-Laryngologica 115:9-17, 1995
Similar abnormal balance tests were common in patients with CFS.

84. Bailey KE, Sloane PD, Mitchell M, Preisser J: Which primary care patients with dizziness will develop persistent impairment? Arch Fam Med 2:847-52, 1993
Certain physical, demographic and preexisting psychological factors are important determinants in whether dizziness will become persistent in primary care patients.

85. Kroenke K, Lucas CA, Rosenberg ML, Scherokman BJ: Psychiatric disorders and functional impairment in patients with persistent dizziness. J Gen Intern Med 8:530-35, 1993
There was a direct relationship of a history of mood disturbances with patients developing persistent dizziness.

86. Goodwin F: A 47-year-old man with chronic depression. JAMA 275:479-85, 1996
A typical case of a patient with depression is discussed with the emphasis on practical management for the primary care physician. There are also important and succinct discussions of drug treatment and the impact of managed health care on mental health treatment.

87. Styron W: Darkness Visible. New York, Vintage Books, 1992
Darkness Visible is Styron's account of his bouts with major depression. It was originally given as a lecture and then expanded to an essay and then to a short book. This quote can be found on page 75.

88. Katon W, Egan K, Miller D: Chronic pain: lifetime psychiatric diagnoses and family history. Am J Psychiatry 142:1156-1159, 1985
Most patients with depression have a history of chronic pain and frequent somatic complaints.

89. Frasure-Smith N, Lesperance F, Talajic M: Depression following myocardial infraction. JAMA 270:1819-1825, 1993
Twenty-five to 50% of people who have a heart attack will also suffer depression during their recuperation. The depression is often unrecognized and very important to treat for an optimal recovery after a heart attack.

90. Eisenberg L: Treating depression and anxiety in primary care. N Engl J Med 326:1080-1084, 1992
Depression and anxiety are often unrecognized and untreated in primary care.

91. Katon W, Sullivan MD: Depression and chronic medical illness. J Clin Psychiatry 52:34-39, 1990
There is a much higher prevalence of depression in patients with chronic medical illnesses than in healthy people. Often the depression is not recognized.

92. Kramer PD: Listening to Prozac. New York, Penguin Books, 1993
Kramer's book made the public very aware of the potential power of the newer, more selective antidepressants, such as Prozac. It also discusses the controversy surrounding the use of such medications in people who do not have major depression but who function better with such medications.

93. Keller MB, Harrison W, Fawcett JA, Geleberg A, Hirschfeld RM, Klein D, Kocsis JH, McCullough JP, Rush AJ, Schatzberg A; Treatment of chronic depression with sertraline or imipramine: preliminary blinded response rates and high rates of undertreatment in the community. Psychopharmacology Bull 31:205-12, 1995
Demonstrated that these antidepressants are effective but not prescribed appropriately.

94. Karp D: Speaking of Sadness. New York, Oxford University Press, 1996
Karp describes his personal and professional experience with depression. He is ambivalent about taking antidepressant medications and viewing depression simply as a disease rather than reflecting a complicated set of social as well as psychological factors.

95. Weil A: Health and Healing. Boston, Houghton Mifflin, 1995
This book is one of the most popular and well-rounded books that deal with non-traditional management of our health. Weil is a physician who has practiced and published extensively on human behavior and development and holistic medicine. The sections of this book on holistic medicine are especially educational.

96. Buchwald D, Garrity D: Comparison of patients with chronic fatigue syndrome, fibromyalgia, and multiple chemical sensitivities. Arch Intern Med 154:2049-2053, 1994
There was striking similarity of demographic features and symptoms in patients with fibromyalgia and chronic fatigue syndrome when compared to those who had been diagnosed with multiple chemical sensitivities.

97. Bohr T: Problems with myofascial pain syndrome and fibromyalgia syndrome. Neurology 46:593-597, 1996
Bohr regards fibromyalgia and the more localized pain disorder, myofascial pain, as nonhistologic aches and pains, given a diagnostic label because of "junk science". He would prefer that terms such as pain amplification syndrome, hypervigilance syndrome or somatoform pain disorder be used. However, our research has demonstrated that the psychiatric diagnosis of somatoform pain disorder is rare in patients with fibromyalgia. Pain amplification implies that patients "amplify their diability and pain", in contrast to "genuine rheumatologic disease, such as rheumatoid arthritis". Bohr further states that certain rheumatologists and attorneys have milked the "cash cow" of fibromyalgia and chronic fatigue syndrome as legal

entities. This personal observation is not based on any research. The vast majority of rheumatologists have avoided litigation issues and have promoted an attitude of encouraging patients with fibromyalgia to stay at work and avoid prolonged disability.

98. Hadler NM: Is fibromyalgia a useful diagnostic label? Cleve Clin J Med 63:85-87, 1996
Hadler calls fibromyalgia a syndrome of "out of sorts". Everyone has bad days that include fatigue, headaches, bowel symptoms and achiness. Depending on the patient's main complaints or the doctor's main interest, these everyday complaints may be labelled as fibromyalgia, chronic fatigue syndrome, irritable bowel syndrome or migraine. The diagnostic labels then "teach the person to be sick". He arguably suggests that the diagnosis of any of these disorder does no good since there is no beneficial therapy and discussion of psychological issues is avoided. However, randomized, clinical trials have demonstrated modest efficacy (certainly equal to that of the treatment of most chronic illnesses) for medicinal and non-medicinal therapies in fibromyalgia. Furthermore, treatment programs in fibromyalgia have been a model of multi-disciplinary "mind-body" management. A number of research studies have documented that applying a diagnostic label to patients with fibromyalgia lessens their symptoms and markedly decreases their use of physicians and hospitals.

99. Awerbuch M: Different concepts of chronic musculoskeletal pain. Ann Rheum Dis 54:331-332, 1995
This editorial uses fibromyalgia, myofascial pain and soft tissue injury as diagnoses of "non-disease". These diagnostic labels are therefore promoting sickness by providing medical authenticity to symptoms and resulting in sympathetic attention, avoidance of unpleasant tasks or work.

100. Abbey SE, Garfinkel PE: Neuasthenia and chronic fatigue syndrome: the role of culture in the making of a diagnosis. Am J Psychiatry 148:1638-1646, 1991

These authors postulate that CFS is the modern-day equivalent to neurasthenia, which was a popular diagnosis in the early 1900s. They suggest that these terms describe psychosocial stress rather than a medical disease.

101. Steiner M, Steinberg S, Stewart D, Carter D, Berger C, Reid R, Grover D, Streiner D: Fluoxetine in the treatment of premenstrual dysphoria. N Eng J Med 332:1529-1534, 1995
Premenstrual dysphoria, often called PMS, causes tension, irritability and depression. Fluoxetine, 20-60 mgs of Prozac, significantly reduced these symptoms in a large group of women with PMS.

102. Cathey MA, Wolfe F, Kleinheksel SM, Hawley DJ: Socioeconomic impact of fibrositis. A study of 81 patients with primary fibrositis. Am J Med 81:78-84, 1986
This study followed a large group of patients with fibrositis (fibromyalgia) and asked questions regarding their health status before and after they were diagnosed and treated. There was less hospitalizations and health care seeking once the diagnosis of fibromyalgia was made.

103. Woodward RV, Broom DH, Legge DG: Diagnosis in chronic illness: disabling or enabling — the case of chronic fatigue syndrome. J R Soc Med 88:325-29, 1995
Discusses the different views of the medical profession and the public regarding a diagnosis of CFS.

104. Brooks PM: Silicone breast implantation: doubts about the fears. Med J Australia 162:432-34, 1995
An overview of the controversy and the lack of science that has been applied.

105. Gabriel SE, O'Fallon WM, Kurland LT, Beard CM, Woods JE, Melton H,III: Risk of connective-tissue disease and other disorders after breast implantation. N Engl J Med 330:1697-1702, 1994
This population study found that women who had received silicone breast implants did not have a significant risk for developing recognized connective tissue disease.

106. Sanchez-Guerrero J, Colditz GA, Karlson EW, Hunter DJ, Speizer FE, Liang MH: Silicone breast implants and the risk of connective-tissue disease and symptoms. N Engl J Med 332:1666-1670, 1995
No significant increased prevalence of connective tissue disorders was found in this large cohort study.

107. Hennekens CH, Lee IM, Cook NR, Hebert PR, Karlson EW, LaMotte F, Manson JE, Buring JE: Self-reported breast implants and connective-tissue diseases in female health professionals. JAMA 275:616-521, 1996
This report also found no large risk of connective tissue disease following breast implants. However, a small increased risk of connective tissue disease could not be excluded.

108. Bridges M, Conley C, Wang G, Burns DE: A clinical and epidemiologic evaluation of women with silicone breast implants and symptoms of rheumatic disease. Ann Intern Med 118:929-936, 1993
Most women who were evaluated for a possible connective tissue disease after receiving a silicone breast implant had nonspecific syndromes, such as fibromyalgia. Some women may have had an ill-defined "new" connective tissue disease.

109. Thomas L: The Medusa and the Snail. New York Viking, 1979
Thomas' writings touch on many topics, mostly medicine and science, but also philosophy and politics.

110. Powell R, Dolan R, Wessely S: Attributions and self-esteem in depression and chronic fatigue syndromes. J Psychosom Res 34:665-673, 1990
Patients with chronic fatigue syndrome who did not attribute their illness to infection or sources outside their influence had a better outcome than those that did.

111. Cluff LE, Canter A, Imboden JB: Asian influenza: infection, disease and psychological factors. Arch Intern Med 117:159-163, 1996

This was one of the earliest studies that demonstrated a relationship of host psychological factors with acquiring and recovering from common viral infections.

112. Frank S, Zyznaski S, Alemagno S: Upper respiratory infection: stress, support, and the medical encounter. Family Med 24:518-523, 1992
A current review of the evidence that stress and support systems have important influences on common respiratory infections.

113. Cohen S, Tyrrell DAJ, Smith AP: Psychological stress and susceptibility to the common cold. N Eng J Med 325:606-612, 1991
Volunteers were inoculated with different viruses that cause colds and upper respiratory infection. The rate that the experimental inoculation produced a clinical infection was directly correlated with the person's preexisting level of stress.

114. Selye H: The general adaptation syndrome and diseases of adaptation. J Clin Endocr 6:117-123, 1946
Selye's landmark studies popularized the notion of a specific physiologic response to stress.

115. Crofford LJ, Demitrack MA: Evidence that abnormalities of central neurohormonal systems are key to understanding fibromyalgia and chronic fatigue syndrome. Rheum Dis Clin N Amer 22:267-284, 1996
Central nervous system aspects of fibromyalgia and CFS are reviewed.

116. Gold PW, Goodwin FK, Chrousos GP: Clinical and biochemical manifestations of depression. Relation to the neurobiology of stress. N Eng J Med 319:348-352, 1988
This article reviews the complicated interactions of the neuroendocrine system and the immune system.

117. Baker GHM, Byrom NA, Irani MS, et al: Stress, cortisol and lymphocyte subpopulations. Lancet 574, 1984

Cortisol production and certain lymphocyte functions are altered by stress.

118. Malarkey WB, Hall JC, Pearl DK, Kiecolt-Glaser JK, Glaser R: The influence of academic stress and season on 24-hour concentrations of growth hormone and prolactin. J Clin Endocrinol Metab 73:1089-1092, 1991
Significant changes in neurohormones, including growth hormone and prolactin, occurred during periods of high academic stress, such as final examinations. Growth hormone and prolactin have been found to be abnormal in some patients with fibromyalgia.

119. Maes M, Bosman E, Suy E, Minner B, Raus J: A further exploration of the relationships between immune parameters and the HPA-axis activity in depressed patients. Psycho Med 21:313-320, 1985
Most studies have demonstrated some alteration of the hypothalamic-pituatary adrenal axis in a subset of patients with major depression.

120. Ader R, Cohen N: Behaviorally conditioned immunosuppression and murine systemic lupus erythematosus. Science 213:1534-1536, 1982
This was one of the most important studies that documented a relationship of the brain to the immune system. Laboratory animals were conditioned to effect their own immune response.

121. Ader R, Cohen N, Felten D: Psychoneuroimmunology interactions between the nervous system and the immune system. Lancet 345:99-103, 1995
This paper reviews the current field of psychoneuroimmunology and potential applications to our health in the future.

122. Crofford LJ, Pillemer SR, Kalogeras KT, Cash JM, Michelson D, Kling MA, Sternberg EM, Gold PW, Chrousos GP, Wilder RL: Hypothalamic-pituitary-adrenal axis perturbations in patients with fibromyalgia. Arthritis Rheum 37:1583-1592, 1994

Abnormalities in neuroendocrine function were found in patients with fibromyalgia. Most investigators have found some alterations in neurohormones in fibromyalgia and CFS although the changes have not been uniform nor present in all patients.

123. Trafford A: The empathy gap. The Washington Post August 29:6, 1995
This newspaper editorial discusses the widening gap between empathy and caring in medicine and high-technology health care.

124. Knox RA: The rust is on in doctors' offices. The Boston Globe March 2:1, 1996
This newspaper feature documents the time pressure that physicians are under as dictated by managed health care.

125. Shore MF, Beigel A: The challenges posed by managed behavioral health care. N Engl J Med 334:116-118, 1996
Managed health care has been especially challenging to the mental health care field. Broad shifts in care, away from long-term psychotherapy to drug treatment and behavioral approaches to mental health, are already in place.

126. Kaplan SH, Greenfield S, Gandek B, Rogers WH, Ware JE: Characteristics of physicians with participatory decision-making styles. Ann Intern Med 124:497-504, 1996
Patients tend to be much more satisfied when their physician allows them to participate in decisions regarding their medical care.

127. Wennberg DE, Kellett MA, Dickens JD, Malenka DJ, Keilson LM, Keller RB: The association between local diagnostic testing intensity and invasive cardiac procedures. JAMA 275:1161-1164, 1996
There was a positive relationship found between the number of stress tests and the number of coronary angiographies and

cardiac revascularizations performed. This study did not determine whether too many invasive studies were being performed. However, the results do indicate that more tests lead to more costly and invasive procedures.

128. Pheasant H, Bursk A, Goldfarb J, Azen SP, Weiss JN, Borelli L: Amitriptyline and chronic low-back pain. A randomized double-blind crossover study. Spine 8: 552-557, 1983
This controlled study demonstrated that amitriptyline was modestly effective in the treatment of chronic, idiopathic low back pain.

129. Cannon RO, Quyyumi AA, Mincemoyer R, Stine AM, et.al.: Imipramine in patients with chest pain despite normal coronary angiograms. N Engl J Med 330:1411-1417, 1994
Ten-30% of patients who undergo coronary angiography for chest pain have normal coronary arteries and are felt to have non-cardiac, visceral pain. Imipramine, another tricyclic medication, at a dose of 50 mg nightly, significantly reduced the pain. The improvement did not correlate with cardiac, esophageal or psychiatric test results.

130. Ades PA, Ballor DL, Ashikaga T, Utton JL, Nair KS: Weight training improves walking endurance in healthy persons. Ann Intern Med 124:568-572, 1996
Weight-training and resistance exercise improved the ability of elderly, well people to walk longer distances.

131. Pioro-Boisset M, Esdaile JM, Fitzcharles M-A: Alternative medicine use in fibromyalgia syndrome. Arthritis Care Res 9:13-17, 1996
Most patients with fibromyalgia had used alternative medicine for their symptoms.

132. Sarno JE: Healing Back Pain. New York, Warner Books, 1991
Sarno has written extensively about back pain. He approaches it from a mind-body view rather than simply a bone or joint structural problem.

133. Fisher P, Greenwood A, Huskisson EC, Turner P, Belon P: Effect of homeopathic treatment on fibrositis (primary fibromyalgia). BMJ 299:365-366, 1989
This controlled study demonstrated some benefit of homeopathy for the treatment of fibromyalgia.

134. Shipley M, Berry H, Broster G, Jenkins M, Clover A, Williams I: Controlled trial of homeopathic treatment of osteoarthritis. Lancet 1:97-98, 1983
Another controlled report demonstrated some improvement when homeopathy was used to treat osteoarthritis.

135. Andrade LE, Ferraz MB, Atra E, Castro A, Silva MS: A randomized controlled trial to evaluate the effectiveness of homeopathy in rheumatoid arthritis. Scand J Rheumatol 20:204-208, 1991
Modest improvement in patients with rheumatoid arthritis was noted in this controlled study of homeopathy.

136. Woolf GM, Petrovic LM, Rojter SE, et al: Acute hepatitis associated with the Chinese herbal product jin bu huan. Ann Intern Med 121:729-735, 1994
A common herbal product produced acute hepatitis.

137. Vanherweghem JL, Depierreux M, Tielemans C, et al: Rapidly progressive interstitial renal fibrosis in young women: association with slimming regimen including chinese herbs. Lancet 341:387-391, 1993
A severe kidney reaction developed in women taking herbal supplements.

138. Roberts IF, West RJ, Ogilvie D, Dillon MJ: Malnutrition in infants receiving cult diets: a form of child abuse. Br Med J 1:296-298, 1979
Cult diets resulted in severe malnutrition in infants. Such dietary approaches to health can cause unforseen morbidity and mortality.

139. Sherlock P, Rothschild EO: Scurvy produced by a Zen macrobiotic diet. JAMA 199:794-798, 1967

A macrobiotic diet was so lacking in vitamin C that it caused scurvey.

140. Carey TS, Garrett J, Jackman A, McLaughlin C, et al: The outcomes and costs of care for acute low back pain among patients seen by primary care practitioners, chiropractors, and orthopedic surgeons. N Engl J Med 333:913-917, 1995
Chiropractic and traditional care were of equal benefit in recovery from low back pain. Chiropractic care was more satisfactory to patients but also cost more than traditional care.

141, Bhatt-Sanders D: Acupuncture for rheumatoid arthritis: an analysis of the literature. Semin Arthritis Rheum 14:225-231, 1985
This study reviews all prior reports of acupuncture for the treatment of rheumatoid arthritis. Few controlled studies have been done.

142. Takeda W, Wessel J: Acupuncture for the treatment of pain of osteoarthritic knees. Arthritis Care Res 7:118-122, 1994
Acupuncture was of some help in the treatment of knee osteoarthritis.

143. Benson H: The Relaxation Response. New York, Morrow, 1975
Benson's work was instrumental in convincing mainstream medicine that the mind and the stress response have important physiologic effects. He studied the effects of relaxation techniques such as meditation on blood pressure and cardiac function.

INDEX

cortisol 42, 116
Crohn's colitis 49
cult diets 148
cyclobenzaprine 18
cyclophosphamide 115
Cytoxan® 115

Dalmane® 45
dehydroepiandrosterone 146
dementia 66
depression 71-80
   association with chronic fatigue 27-28
   diagnosis 73-74
   symptoms 71-72
   treatment 77-80
DHEA 146
digitalis 143
Diseases 1-5
   diagnosis 1-2, 10, 12
   medical model of 7
   risk factors of 4
   vs. illness 4-5, 10, 21
dizziness 27, 67-68, 86
dysthymia 73

Eastern medicine 112, 138, 143-144
Effexor® 27
Elavil® 18
electrical stimulation 137, 149
elimination diet 90-91
endorphins 136
energy healing 141
environment 2, 77, 84, 88-91
eosinophilia-myalgia syndrome 145
epinephrine 116
Epstein-Barr virus 24, 90-91
ergonomics 138
ergot derivatives 131